Paediatric Dentistry at a Glance

Titles in the dentistry *At a Glance* series

Paediatric Dentistry at a Glance

Monty Duggal BDS, MDS, FDS (Paeds), RCS (Eng), PhD
Professor and Head of Paediatric Dentistry
Department of Paediatric Dentistry
Leeds Dental Institute
Leeds
UK

Angus Cameron BDS, MDSc, FDSRCS (Eng), FRACDS, FICD
Head of Department, Paediatric Dentistry and Orthodontics
Westmead Hospital
and
Clinical Associate Professor and Head, Paediatric Dentistry
The University of Sydney
NSW
Australia

Jack Toumba BSc (Hons), BChD, MSc, FDS (Paeds), RCS (Eng), PhD
Professor of Paediatric and Preventive Dentistry
Department of Paediatric Dentistry
Leeds Dental Institute
Leeds
UK

WILEY-BLACKWELL
A John Wiley & Sons, Ltd., Publication

This edition first published 2013
© 2013 by John Wiley & Sons Ltd.

Wiley-Blackwell is an imprint of John Wiley & Sons, formed by the merger of Wiley's global Scientific, Technical and Medical business with Blackwell Publishing.

Registered office: John Wiley & Sons, Ltd, The Atrium, Southern Gate, Chichester, West Sussex, PO19 8SQ, UK

Editorial offices: 9600 Garsington Road, Oxford, OX4 2DQ, UK

The Atrium, Southern Gate, Chichester, West Sussex, PO19 8SQ, UK

2121 State Avenue, Ames, Iowa 50014-8300, USA

For details of our global editorial offices, for customer services and for information about how to apply for permission to reuse the copyright material in this book please see our website at www.wiley.com/wiley-blackwell.

Library of Congress Cataloging-in-Publication Data

Duggal, Monty S.
   Paediatric dentistry at a glance / Monty Duggal, Angus Cameron, Jack Toumba.
      p. ; cm. – (At a glance series)
   Includes bibliographical references and index.
   ISBN 978-1-4443-3676-4 (pbk. : alk. paper)
   I. Cameron, Angus C.   II. Toumba, Jack.   III. Title.   IV. Series: At a glance series (Oxford, England)
   [DNLM: 1. Dental Care for Children–Handbooks.   2. Child–Handbooks.   3. Tooth Diseases–Handbooks.   WU 49]

   617.6'45–dc23

2012015790

A catalogue record for this book is available from the British Library.

Wiley also publishes its books in a variety of electronic formats. Some content that appears in print may not be available in electronic books.

Cover image: courtesy of the authors
Cover design by Meaden Creative

Set in 9/11.5 pt Times by Toppan Best-set Premedia Limited
Printed in Singapore by Ho Printing Singapore Pte Ltd

1   2013

Contents

1 Planning treatment for children

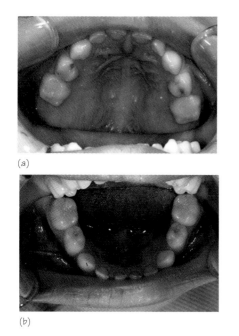

(a)

(b)

Figure 1.1 Intra-oral view showing the carious upper (a) and lower (b) primary molars.

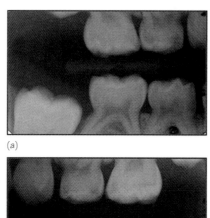

(a)

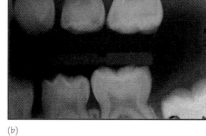

(b)

Figure 1.2 Bitewing radiographs showing extent of caries.

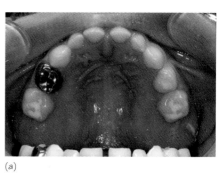

(a)

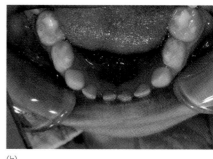

(b)

Figure 1.3 Intra-oral view showing upper (a) and lower (b) arches at the end of treatment.

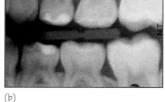

(a)   (b)

Figure 1.4 Postoperative radiographs of the treated case.

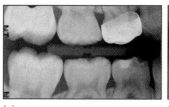

(a)   (b)

Figure 1.5 Follow-up visit revealed that first permanent molars had erupted and these were fissure sealed.

Table 1.1 Step-by-step plan of the proposed treatment where prevention is carried out alongside restorative care.

Visit	Treatment	Preventative
One	Examination and treatment plan Correspondence with paediatrician	Oral hygiene instructions Use of adult tooth paste Diet sheet was given
Two	Full mouth prophylaxis 55 – Fissure sealant 65 – Fissure sealant 75 – Fissure sealant 85 – Fissure sealant Temporisation of 54 and 64	Reinforce oral hygiene instructions Collect diet sheet Duraphat™ (22 600 ppm F) Plaque score
Three	64 – Composite restoration	Reinforce oral hygiene measures Diet counselling Duraphat™ (22 600 ppm F)
Four	54 – Stainless steel crown	Reinforce diet advice Plaque score Duraphat™ (22 600 ppm F)
Five	74 – Composite restoration	Reinforce oral hygiene measures

Paediatric Dentistry at a Glance, First Edition. Monty Duggal, Angus Cameron and Jack Toumba. © 2013 John Wiley & Sons Ltd. Published 2013 by Blackwell Publishing Ltd.

General philosophy of the authors

Dentists who treat children are in a unique position not only to provide dental treatment when required, but to influence the future behaviour, attitudes to oral health and attitude towards dentistry in general. Children deserve the highest quality care and highest quality restorative dentistry should be provided to them, supplemented with rigorous prevention. Prevention of dental caries in children should be a priority but sadly nearly half of 5-year-olds, even in developed countries, still develop dental caries. A non-interventionist approach, as has been advocated in some countries such as the UK, or poor restorative patchwork dentistry, is doomed to failure and only leads to pain, infection and suffering in children, requiring more invasive interventions. These are traumatic and expensive and negatively influence the child's future behaviour and attitudes to dentistry. Good restorative and preventive care obviates the need for extraction of primary teeth under general anaesthesia, a practice which should have only a small place in the dental care of young children. In addition, in a developing child, the dentist has the task of monitoring the dentition, diagnosis and management of anomalies as well as having a knowledge of medical conditions and the provision of safe restorative care for children.

Philosophy of treatment planning

- Gain the trust and cooperation of the child.
- Make an accurate diagnosis and devise a treatment plan appropriate to the child's need.
- Comprehensive preventive care.
- Deliver care in a manner the child finds acceptable.
- Use materials and techniques which provide effective and long-lasting results.

History

This should include medical history, social history, history of the present complaint and the past dental history. What were the "likes" and "dislikes" of the child at previous dental visits? In addition, parents' assessment of the previous and expected child's behaviour is useful.

Examination

- A good examination using tell–show–do, including charting for teeth present and caries, including areas of early decalcification.
- Any missing teeth.
- Gingival health.
- Developmental defects.
- Tooth surface loss.
- Initial occlusal assessment.

Radiographs and other investigations

Appropriate radiographs such as bitewings or OPG (Chapter 10) or any other special tests such as pulp sensibility tests.

Diagnosis

In children the diagnosis needs to encompass two aspects:
- diagnosis of the dental/oral condition;
- the child's behaviour and the behavioural approach likely to succeed in provision of the treatment.

Diagnosis should be specific. For example, a diagnosis "dental caries" in itself is incomplete as it does not specify the reason the child has dental caries. The root cause of the problem cannot be addressed unless a specific diagnosis is made.

Formulating treatment plan

An example of a treated case and the step-by-step treatment plan is shown is Figs. 1.1–1.5 and Table 1.1 respectively. When managing caries in children this should relate to:
- prognosis of the affected teeth;
- child's behaviour and likely acceptance of the treatment.

Restore or extract

- Extent of caries. Are the teeth restorable?
- Impact that either option will have not only on developing dentition but child's long-term well-being.
- When all primary molars are involved, give consideration to restoring the second and extraction of the first primary molars.

Each treatment plan should be tailor-made for the child. For some children, comprehensive restorative care using one of the behavioural approaches is appropriate. For others extraction of some primary teeth and restoration of the others with local analgesia (LA) or general anaesthesia (GA) is more appropriate.

Management strategy – LA, LA with sedation or GA?

Most children are amenable to behaviour guidance. However, when planning treatment, the child's well-being, and also the impact that multiple visits of invasive treatment under local analgesia might have on the child's future behaviour and attitude towards dental treatment should be considered. Access to good GA facilities is essential.

Preventive strategy

Depending on the caries risk, a preventive strategy is devised.

Choice of materials

This depends on tooth to be restored, past caries history and cooperation of the child. An important consideration in children is that the tooth should only need restoring once. In very young children where a restoration is required to last 4–5 years, due consideration should be given to the use of stainless steel crowns.

Developmental anomalies

Formulate a short-, medium- and long-term plan.

Medical history and treatment planning

- Liaise with medical practitioner.
- Understand the impact of the medical condition on the provision of treatment.

In the following chapters all the aspects that play a role in the management of children's oral and dental health are discussed.

2 Growth and development

Table 2.1 Growth period. Lowrey's classification (1973).

Growth period	Chronological age
Prenatal	Conception to birth (40 weeks)
Infancy	Birth to 2 years
Early childhood (preschool)	3–6 years Toddlers – second and third year Play stage – 4–6 years
Late childhood (prepubertal)	7–12 years Puberty age range for girls 10–14 years, puberty age range for boys 12–16 years
Adolescence	13–20 years

Table 2.2 Disturbances in prenatal development.

Genetic disturbances	Environmental disturbances
Chromosomal: Down syndrome, chromosome 18 Polygenic (several genes), e.g. cleft lip/palate Monogenic (single gene), e.g. enzyme deficiencies, amelogenesis imperfecta, chondrodysplasia, some craniofacial syndromes	Medication: thalidomide Maternal infections: rubella, toxoplasmosis X-ray radiation Anorexia Maternal malnutrition Maternal alcoholism

Table 2.3 Disturbances in postnatal development.

Primary	Secondary
Skeletal dysplasias – 100 disorders where genetic damage or defect to skeletal system Chromosomal aberrations/disorders, e.g. Down syndrome, Turner's syndrome Congenital errors of metabolism, e.g. mucopolysaccharidoses (genetic conditioned failures in the intercellular substance in the connective tissues), Hunter syndrome, Hurler syndrome Miscellaneous syndromes. Unknown aetiology but seen at birth Genetic short stature (familial)	Malnutrition: if prolonged and severe. Poverty and poor nutrition. Emotional and physical abuse Systemic and metabolic disorders, e.g. coeliac disease, cystic fibrosis, chronic renal disease Deprivation dwarfism (psychosocial growth retardation), caused by disturbances in emotional contact between child, parents and environment Endocrine disorders: growth, sex or thyroid hormone deficiency, hypothyroidism Constitutional growth delay and puberty (normal variant): children with delayed skeletal maturity. They tend to have delayed growth and sexual maturation but their final height will be normal

Paediatric Dentistry at a Glance, First Edition. Monty Duggal, Angus Cameron and Jack Toumba. © 2013 John Wiley & Sons Ltd. Published 2013 by Blackwell Publishing Ltd.

Development of the nasomaxillary complex
- Grows downwards and forwards relative to the cranial base and greatest during pubertal growth spurt.
- Areas near sutures found at maxilla and cranial base have bone deposition as brain grows and soft tissue of face forms.
- During pubertal growth spurt, facial skeleton growth starts and is almost completed at age 15.5 years in girls and later in boys.

Mandibular growth
- Greatest during pubertal growth spurt.
- Growth of mandible coordinates with growth of maxilla and cranial base in forward and downward direction (translation of the mandible).
- Bony deposition at ramus and in condyles allows mandible to grow downwards and forward.
- Mandibular condylar cartilage (reactive growth site) is involved in bone formation with cartilage proliferation and its replacement by bone.

Tooth development
Teeth start to form very early on, around the 5th week of the embryo. The dental lamina gives rise to epithelial buds that then differentiate into the tooth germ, within which reside the cells for the development of the various tooth structures. The odontoblasts form dentine and ameloblasts form the enamel. The epithelial structure known as the root sheath of Hertwig arises from an apical migration of the epithelial cells at the cervical loop of the enamel organ and is responsible for the development of the roots of the teeth.

Tooth eruption
Eruption times for the primary teeth (in months)
Lower central incisor: 7–8
Upper incisors: 10–11
Upper lateral: 11
Lower lateral: 13
First primary molars: 16
Canines: 19
Second primary molars: 27–29

Eruption times permanent dentition (in years)
First molar and lower central incisor: 6
Upper central and lower lateral incisors: 7
Upper lateral incisor: 8
Lower canines and first premolars: 10
Upper canine and second premolars: 11
Second molars: 12
Third molars: 16 onwards

Methods of assessing growth
The growth periods as described by Lowrey (1973) are shown in Table 2.1.

- Chronological age.
- Neurological age.
- Morphological age.
- Skeletal age.
- Mental age.
- Secondary sex characteristics.
- Dental age.

Methods of monitoring somatic growth
- Length/height.
- Weight.
- Head circumference.
- Behavioural milestones.
- Dental age.

Height and weight are usually monitored using standard growth charts. For height the most common one used is height velocity chart and for weight the BMI-for-age chart.

Dental age – why is it important?
Dental age correlates well with chronological age. It is important for dentists to have a knowledge of growth and development, especially of the dentition, for the following reasons:
- tooth eruption sequence is important – if any problems with the occlusion occur, it is important to check whether the eruption sequence is correct, especially in cases where teeth might be developmentally absent;
- tooth emergence dates are used in orthodontics for timing of treatment;
- timing of fluoride supplements (systemic fluoride) depends on the dental age (prevention advice);
- stages of development are important when considering loss of the permanent first molars;
- stage of apical development in incisors is important in cases of trauma to monitor pulp healing.

It is also important for paediatric dentists to understand the difference in growth between males and females to help in the management of the developing dentition and provision of interceptive orthodontic care:
- growth in height between boys and girls is almost parallel up to age 10 years;
- in girls, age 11–13 years, female oestrogens causes rapid growth and bony epiphyses uniting at age 14–16 years;
- in boys, testosterone causes later prolonged growth (age 13–17 years).

Disturbances in prenatal and postnatal development are shown in Tables 2.2 and 2.3.

Child cognitive and psychological development

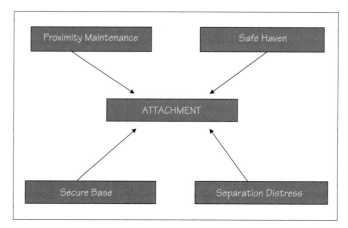

Figure 3.1 Characteristics of attachment according to John Bowlby (1969).

Table 3.1 Erikson's psychosocial theory – stages of development and crisis/conflicts at each stage.

Stages	Crisis or conflict
Stage 1	Trust vs mistrust
Stage 2	Autonomy vs shame or guilt
Stage 3	Initiative vs guilt
Stage 4	Industry vs inferiority
Stage 5	Identity vs confusion
Stage 6	Intimacy vs isolation
Stage 7	Generativity vs stagnation
Stage 8	Integrity vs despair

Paediatric Dentistry at a Glance, First Edition. Monty Duggal, Angus Cameron and Jack Toumba. © 2013 John Wiley & Sons Ltd. Published 2013 by Blackwell Publishing Ltd.

Introduction

In order to understand behaviour management for helping children accept dental care, a basic knowledge of the child's cognitive and psychological development is essential.

Theories of cognitive and psychological development

The cognitive capability of children changes from birth through to adulthood. Various theories divide this process into a number of stages for clarity and ease of description.

John Piaget's theory of cognitive development

This important theory has three important concepts, schema, assimilation and accommodation. Schemas are categories of knowledge that help us to interpret and understand the world. The process of taking in new information into our previously existing schemas is known as assimilation. Accommodation involves altering existing schemas, or ideas, as a result of new information or new experiences.

Piaget believed that all children try to strike a balance between assimilation and accommodation, which is achieved through a mechanism called equilibration. As children progress through the stages of cognitive development, it is important to maintain a balance between applying previous knowledge (assimilation) and changing behaviour to account for new knowledge (accommodation). Equilibration helps explain how children are able to move from one stage of thought into the next.

According to Piaget there are four stages of cognitive development:

1. sensorimotor period;
2. preoperational period;
3. concrete operational stage;
4. formal operational period.

Erikson's psychosocial theory (Table 3.1)

Erikson believed that personality develops in stages with each stage characterised by a conflict or a crisis (Table 3.1). The stages are:

- Stage 1. Infancy: age 0–1 years.
- Stage 2. Toddler: age 1–2 years.
- Stage 3. Early childhood: age 2–6 years.
- Stage 4. Elementary and middle school years: age 6–12 years.
- Stage 5. Adolescence: age 12–18 years.
- Stage 6, 7 and 8 relate to young adulthood through late adulthood.

Freud's psychosexual theory

Freud's theory stressed the importance of childhood events and experiences, but are focused almost solely on mental disorders rather than normal functioning. For this reason this is of limited importance for paediatric dentists, but is discussed here for the sake of completeness.

- Oral stage. Age 0–1.5 years.
- Anal stage. Age 1.5–3 years.
- Phallic stage. Age 4–5 years.
- Latency. Age 5 years to puberty.
- Genital stage. Puberty onwards.

Behavioural theories of child development

1. Classical conditioning by Pavlov. This is learning through association. The theory is based on conditioned and unconditioned stimulus and response. An unconditioned stimulus unconditionally and automatically triggers a response. A conditioned stimulus is one that is previously a neutral stimulus but after becoming associated with the unconditioned stimulus, eventually comes to trigger a conditioned response, which is learned.

2. Operant conditioning by Skinner. This is learning through consequences. The term **operant** refers to any "active behaviour that operates upon the environment to generate consequences". This is a method of learning that is possible through rewards and punishments for behaviour. Through this form of conditioning, an association is made between behaviour and a consequence for that behaviour. This theory is of great significance in paediatric dentistry as it is the basis of the behaviour management technique called behaviour shaping. It has three main principles:

- **Reinforcement**: a consequence that causes behaviour to occur with greater frequency in future. Positive reinforcement is the addition of a favourable, pleasant stimulus following behaviour, such as praise or giving a small gift, for example stickers. Negative reinforcement is the removal of an aversive, unpleasant stimulus following behaviour.
- **Punishment**: a consequence that causes behaviour to occur with less frequency in the future. Positive punishment can be administered through the addition of an unpleasant stimulus following behaviour whereas negative punishment implies the removal of a pleasant stimulus following behaviour.
- **Extinction** is the lack of any consequences following behaviour. Such an inconsequential behaviour will occur with less frequency in future.

3. Observational learning. Learning by observation. It does not require direct personal experience with stimuli, reinforcers or punishers. Children learn by simply watching the behaviour of another person called a model and later imitating the model's behaviour. This technique is used often to manage behaviour of children in paediatric dentistry.

Social theories of child development

The attachment theory by John Bowlby (Fig. 3.1)

Child development is best understood within the framework of patterns of interaction between the child and the primary caregiver. If there were problems in this relationship then the child is likely to form insecure and anxious patterns. According to Bowlby there are four characteristics of attachment:

- **proximity maintenance** – the desire to be near the people we are attached to;
- **safe haven** – returning to the attachment figure for comfort and safety in the face of a fear or threat;
- **secure base** – the attachment figure acts as a base of security from which the child can explore the surrounding environment;
- **separation distress** – anxiety that occurs in the absence of the attachment figure.

Vygotsky's sociocultural theory

Sociocultural theory stresses the important contributions that society makes to individual development. Cognitive growth and complex thinking evolve out of social interactions. An important concept of this theory is the "zone of proximal development", which stresses the ability of the child to learn under guidance and knowledge and skills that a person cannot yet understand or perform on their own yet, but is capable of learning through collaboration with more capable peers.

4 Behaviour management

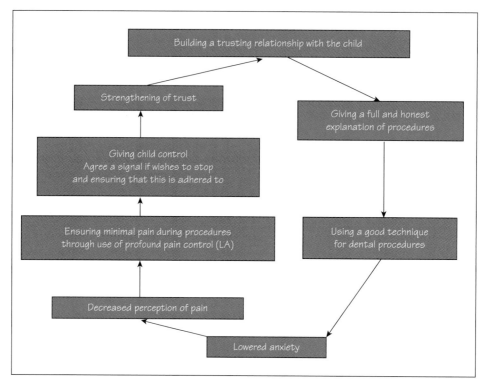

Figure 4.1 Building a relationship between child and dentist (adapted from Feigal, 2001).

Table 4.1 Some "child-friendly" terms used to describe dental equipment and procedures.

Slow speed hand piece	Buzzy bee
Air rotor	Whizzy brush, tooth shower, Mr Whistle
Air spray, Inhalation sedation	Magic air/wind
Local anaesthetic	Jungle juice, sleepy juice, putting tooth to sleep
Rubber dam	Raincoat
Suction	Hoover

Paediatric Dentistry at a Glance, First Edition. Monty Duggal, Angus Cameron and Jack Toumba. © 2013 John Wiley & Sons Ltd. Published 2013 by Blackwell Publishing Ltd.

Introduction

Helping the child to accept dental treatment without a negative experience that might influence the way the child views dental treatment and consequently dental health in the future is one of the most important skills that a paediatric dentist must learn.

The successful management of children in dentistry is a team effort with the parent, the dentist, the dental team and the ambience of the clinical environment all playing their part.

Dentist's manner and appearance

A paediatric dentist must like children for a start and be able to communicate at the level of the child's understanding. Ideas and concepts have to be broken down in terms understood by the child. The use of "childrenese" terms helps explain dental instruments and procedures in a non-threatening manner that is acceptable to most children. Genuine interest in the child's welfare can be transferred to the child and help them feel more secure and safe. Some personality types are able to do this naturally without thinking, whilst others may have to learn these skills.

It seems that the dentist's attire is not as important as general cleanliness and neatness. Personal hygiene is most important. However, some children do suffer from "white-coat" syndrome and a dentist wearing child-friendly attire may help alleviate some anxiety.

Protective equipment like facemasks and goggles are accepted well by the patients if worn after a brief explanation of their roles and function. They have less influence on subsequent behaviour.

Building trust with the child and empathy are two most important basic principles of the successful management of a child in a dental environment (Fig. 4.1). A trusting relationship with the dentist increases the child's acceptance of dental procedures and the success of treatment will further strengthen trust and rapport.

The dental environment

The clinical area for children should be designed to put children at ease. It should be carefully designed, welcoming, appear non-threatening and safe, yet able to function clinically.

Parental and peer influences

Parents' and peers' attitude to dental treatment has a profound influence on the child. Although the parent must have an active and valued role in the child's oral health, their presence in the surgery can pose a challenge for the dentist, especially if the parent feels that they have to be involved in verbal communication with the child during treatment. There is no clear evidence on whether the parent is in or out of the surgery has any influence on the child's behaviour. The following circumstances for inclusion of the parent are now generally accepted by paediatric dentists:

- all pre-school children;
- children with physical, emotional or psychological impairments;
- children having an examination carried out (for consent purposes, especially for radiographs);
- when the parent and/or patient expressly wish for the parent to remain present.

However, whether the parent stays in or out is a very much an individual decision based on the preference of the dentist, child and parent.

Basic behaviour management techniques

Basic behaviour management or guidance strategies based on positive reinforcement include:

- tell–show–do;
- behaviour shaping;
- modelling;
- distraction.

All these techniques are underpinned by effective communication, voice modulation and making the child feel in control of the treatment. Voice modulation is learnt through experience, and the purpose is to affect the behaviour with subtle changes in the volume, tone or pace of the verbal instruction, without any hint of anger or annoyance. Asking the child to raise their hand if they feel uncomfortable and wish for you to stop is effective in making the child feel in control. However, if this instruction is given and the child does raise the hand, the dentist must stop, otherwise it can lead to a breach of trust between the child and the dentist.

Tell–show–do

This forms the basis for most behaviour guidance strategies in the clinic. A short explanation of the next step before introducing it, rather than the other way around, prepares the child and improves the acceptance of the procedure. Some child-friendly terms for description of the dental procedures and equipment are shown in Table 4.1.

Behaviour shaping

This is based on Skinner's theory of operant conditioning and positive reinforcement is an important element of this technique. The dental procedure is introduced in small steps, the least anxiety provoking first, and upon acceptance positive reinforcement is provided to the child. A simple "well done", "your mum/dad are really proud of you" or "you are so brave/good" usually works well. Through a series of such approximations each followed by a positive reinforcement, the desired behaviour is achieved. A reward, such as a sticker or a small soft toy at the end of a visit, provided the child has done well, is also an effective reinforcement. No reward should be made if the visit has not gone well, especially if the child has behaved badly, as this just reinforces bad behaviour.

Modelling

Other children in the surgery can serve as models, whilst they are having dental procedures being carried out. Alternatively video clips of other children having dental treatment playing on TV monitors can also help.

Distraction

Various types of activities can be used to distract the child's attention. Playing appropriate movies, playing on video games etc. can be useful. However, in the authors' opinion, talking to the child throughout treatment is an effective method of achieving this aim.

5 Aversive conditioning and management of phobia

Box 5.1 A suggested hierarchy for carrying out systematic desensitisation to achieve local analgesia in those who are needle phobic

1. Instructions on relaxation breathing or administration of inhalation sedation
2. Explain the components of LA equipment
3. Allow patient to look at dental syringe from a distance
4. Show and explain topical analgesia
5. Explain factually how LA is administered
6. Encourage patient to hold syringe in hand
7. Encourage patient to hold syringe against cheek
8. Hold syringe with needle guard and against mucosa
9. Press syringe against mucosa
10. Apply topical anaesthetic
11. Remove guard and hold syringe without needle guard against mucosa gently
12. Penetrate the mucosa gently without delivering any anaesthetic solution until patient is relaxed
13. Deliver a minute amount of solution very gently and assess patient's relaxation
14. Continue slowly using positive reinforcement

Box 5.2 Development of fear

1. **Classical conditioning (direct pathway)**
   - Children who had negative experiences associated with medical treatment may be more anxious about dental treatment (Wright *et al.*, 1971)
   - Fear sustained from previous unhappy dental visits has also been related to poor behaviour at subsequent visits

2. **Modelling (indirect pathway)**
   - Acquired fears from parents, peers, siblings
   - Relationship between maternal dental anxiety and difficulties in child patient management at all ages has been shown (Freeman, 1999) and is particularly important for children less than 4 years old

3. **Information/instruction (indirect pathway)**
   - From school, media, friends

4. **Intellectual capacities**
   - Depend on age and psychological development
   - Children with communication or learning difficulties

5. **Dispositional factors**
   - Child's coping style, values
   - Child's age. Highest level of dental anxiety usually at 4 years of age and an overall decrease appears as children become older
   - Child's familial situation (parents' divorce)

6. **Environmental factors and dental surgery**
   - Dental setting; colours, smell, sounds
   - Time of the appointment
   - Dentist's appearance (white coat phobia) and behaviour (verbal and non-verbal communication)
   - Dental staff's appearance and behaviour
   - Appearance and sounds of dental devices and rotary instruments
   - Non-dental chat between dentist and nurse, dentist and parents

Paediatric Dentistry at a Glance, First Edition. Monty Duggal, Angus Cameron and Jack Toumba. © 2013 John Wiley & Sons Ltd. Published 2013 by Blackwell Publishing Ltd.

Introduction

Many children who are either too anxious, used to having their own way at home or harbour genuine phobia regarding various aspects of dental treatment, require more specialised approaches to management. For this reason an understanding of the theories of learning and development is important and will help the dentist not only to provide the immediate care that the child requires but also help shape the child's positive attitude for future dental treatment.

Aversive conditioning

Aversive conditioning is a form of behaviour therapy in which an aversive stimulus, which is an object or event that causes strong feelings of dislike or disgust, is paired with an undesirable behaviour in order to reduce or eliminate that undesirable behaviour.

The purpose of aversive conditioning is to decrease or eliminate undesirable behaviours and it focuses on changing a specific behaviour in order to bring out changes. In such situations, both the type of behaviour and the type of aversive stimulus used will influence the treatment that is being undertaken.

In aversive conditioning negative reinforcement is deployed.

Negative reinforcement

Negative reinforcement procedure consists of presenting a stimulus until a response is performed that removes or reduces the effects of a stimulus. This is not to be confused with punishment, because the removal of the negative reinforcement strengthens the desired behaviour.

Behaviour modification strategies

Aversive conditioning and negative reinforcement are usually employed in situations where all other avenues to establish communication with the child have been exhausted. These approaches are not used again and again in the same child but on one occasion to establish communication, following which conventional techniques based on positive reinforcement are introduced.

Flooding

Flooding is defined as a type of desensitisation for the treatment of phobias without being able to escape until the lack of reinforcement of the anxiety response causes its extinction. Essentially, flooding is "exposure treatment" where the patient is exposed to their greatest fear but are not in danger or harmed in any way. A simple example is to help the child confront their fears of sitting in the dental chair, the child is lifted and placed in the dental chair which allows the child to realise that this was not so threatening after all.

Selective exclusion of the parent

When the child exhibits tantrum behaviour and communication between dentist and child is lost, the parent is requested by the dentist to leave the treatment room. Before this is done a full explanation should be provided to the parent, who must agree to comply. Also, the child must be told the conditions for the recall of the parent before they are sent out. Once the desired behaviour is exhibited, the parent is recalled into the surgery, which being the negative reinforcement will strengthen the desired behaviour.

Phobia

Phobia should be distinguished from anxiety.

Dental anxiety is a state of apprehension regarding the dental treatment. It is normal for people to be anxious regarding situations which are perceived to be pain invoking. **Dental phobia**, on the other hand, is an irrational, intense, persistent fear of certain aspects of dental treatment, such as needle phobia.

Dental anxiety is managed by the traditional behaviour guidance strategies, but the management of severe anxiety, and in particular needle phobia requires special techniques, such as systematic desensitisation.

Systematic desensitisation

This is a type of behavioural therapy introduced by Joseph Wolpe (1969) based on the understanding that relaxation and anxiety cannot exist at the same time in an individual. In practice, for the management of dental phobia, a hierarchy of fear-producing stimuli is constructed and the patient is exposed to them in an ordered manner, starting with the stimulus posing the lowest threat. However, before this is done, the patient is taught to relax; only when a state of relaxation is achieved, the fear-provoking stimuli are introduced hierarchically with the least fear-provoking introduced first and only progressing to the next when the patient feels able. Often, inhalation sedation is used to induce a state of relaxation where systematic desensitisation is planned. A protocol that has been suggested in the literature is shown in Box 5.1.

One of the key elements of systematic desensitisation is inducing a state of relaxation, which may take several visits to achieve. Particularly in adolescents where the anxiety about the needle is deep and intense, but not a phobia, a technique also known as rapid desensitisation can be used. After induction of a state of relaxation, the patient is introduced to the anxiety-provoking stimuli quite quickly, one after another in the same visit, in order to achieve treatment in that visit. However, this may not be possible in those who have genuine needle phobia.

Special devices for delivery of local analgesia, such as the Wand, can also be used, as the patient may have had no previous exposure to these and they would therefore not be anxiety provoking. This will be discussed in Chapter 6.

Preventing the development of dental phobia

Clinicians should make every effort to reduce fear in children during dental treatment. It is not always possible for all procedures to be painless, or totally comfortable for the child. However, through good communication, empathy and a sound knowledge of behaviour-guidance strategies, it is possible to prepare children to accept uncomfortable procedures without negatively affecting their view of dental treatment, and through that the importance of good dental health. Box 5.2 summarises the current understanding of how fear develops in children.

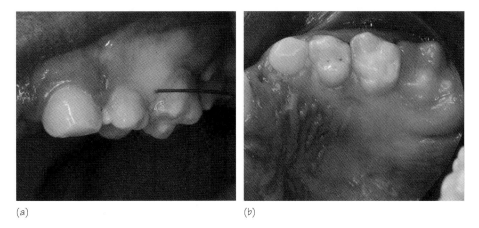

(a) (b)

Figure 6.1 Indirect palatal analgesia is achieved by injecting through the already anaesthetised buccal papilla.

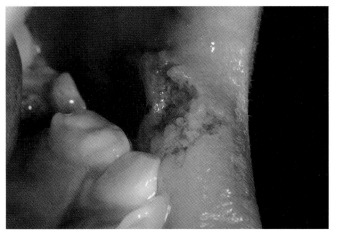

Figure 6.2 Lip injury inflicted by the child chewing the lip after an IDB. Children and parents must be given clear postoperative instructions after administration of an IDB.

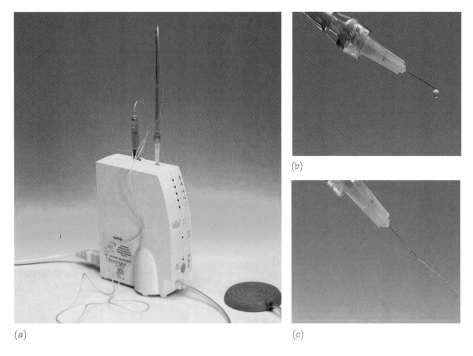

(a) (b) (c)

Figure 6.3 (a) Wand. The speed of delivery can be controlled to be either slow (b) in anxious patients or faster (c) by applying the correct pressure on the foot pedal.

Paediatric Dentistry at a Glance, First Edition. Monty Duggal, Angus Cameron and Jack Toumba. © 2013 John Wiley & Sons Ltd. Published 2013 by Blackwell Publishing Ltd.

Philosophy

Many dentists are reluctant to administer an "injection" to children for dental treatment and feel that they can undertake restorative treatment in children without the use of local analgesia. This is a myth, and in the authors' view it is not possible to achieve good quality restorative dentistry in children without local analgesia. It is incumbent on all those who treat children to do so with adequate pain control.

Explanation

The full procedure should be explained to the child in simple terms, such as "putting the tooth to sleep" or putting "jungle juice" around the tooth. A signal should be agreed with the child whereby they can indicate when they are feeling uncomfortable, such as putting their hand up to indicate discomfort.

Topical/surface analgesia

A flavoured topical analgesic should always be used. The most commonly used is topical 20% benzocaine, which is available in various flavours.

1. Apply in small quantity on cotton roll or cotton bud.
2. Ensure that area of application is dry to avoid it leecing into saliva as the taste might then upset some children.
3. Apply for at least 1 minute for best effect.

Commonly used local anaesthetics

• Lignocaine 2% with 1:80000 epinephrine.
• Prilocaine 3% with felypressin 0.54 µg/ml.
• Articaine 4% with 1:100000 epinephrine.

Lignocaine 2% with epinephrine remains the most commonly used anaesthetic solution in dentistry. However, in the last few years the use of articaine has increased. There is some limited evidence that in young children infiltration with 4% articaine with 1:100000 epinephrine gives as profound an analgesia as inferior dental block (IDB) with lignocaine for the restoration of mandibular posterior teeth, including for pulp therapy in primary molars. In the authors' opinion it certainly seems to give profound analgesia with mandibular infiltration and with careful case selection can be used instead of an IDB in many cases.

Infiltration analgesia

• Most frequently used for restorative procedures in maxillary teeth and for minor soft tissue surgical procedures such as removal of mucocoele, epulis etc.
• Lignocaine used as infiltration does not reliably provide profound analgesia for mandibular teeth especially for procedures involving the pulp. Articaine works better.

Direct/indirect palatal

Required for:
• extractions of maxillary teeth;
• securing palatal analgesia for placement of rubber dam clamp in maxillary teeth.

In most cases a full palatal injection is not required. An indirect palatal injection can be given through the buccal papilla after administering buccal infiltration. The needle is advanced through to just below the palatal mucosa where the solution is deposited to secure palatal analgesia (Fig. 6.1). Also can be referred to as transpapillary injection.

Inferior dental block

• Required for most mandibular primary molars requiring pulpal analgesia.
• Supplemented by a long buccal infiltration when placing rubber dam clamp or for extractions of mandibular teeth.

In children this gives a feeling of profound numbness of the lip on the same side. Children and parents should be warned regarding this and child warned not to bite, chew or suck the lip or cheek (Fig. 6.2).

Intraligamental

• Seldom required for primary teeth due to a small risk of damage to permanent tooth germ.
• Very effective to supplement other techniques especially where it is proving difficult to achieve analgesia. Examples are hypersensitive carious exposed pulps in young permanent molars, hypomineralised permanent molars, or for extraction of permanent molars where other forms of analgesia have failed.

Although many commercial syringes are available for this, the use of the Wand for intraligamental analgesia is the best and least painful method.

The Wand (Fig. 6.3)

This is a computerised delivery system based on two principles:
• slow delivery, the speed of which can be controlled with a foot pedal;
• extra-fine needle designed to be inserted with rotatory movement.
  The Wand is particularly useful in children in the following situations:
• children who had a previous bad experience with conventional injection and associate a syringe with pain;
• for intraligamental analgesia as the extra fine needle and slow delivery help reduce discomfort.

Contraindications of local analgesia

• Bleeding disorders. Block contraindicated except with appropriate factor replacement.
• Injection at infection site. Block analgesia or intraligamental might be effective in this situation.
• Malignant hyperpyrexia. Pre-treatment with dantrolene sodium may be required, seek medical advice.
• Known allergy to the LA drug.
• Use with caution in liver and renal dysfunction.

Maximum doses

These are shown in Table 6.1.

Table 6.1 Maximum doses of commonly used local analgesic preparations.

Drug	Without vasoconstrictor	With vasoconstrictor
2% lignocaine	4.4 mg/kg	6.6 mg/kg
4%/3% prilocaine	8.0 mg/kg	6.0 mg/kg
3%/2% mepivicaine	6.6 mg/kg	6.6 mg/kg
4% articaine	7.0 mg/kg	7.0 mg/kg

7 Conscious sedation

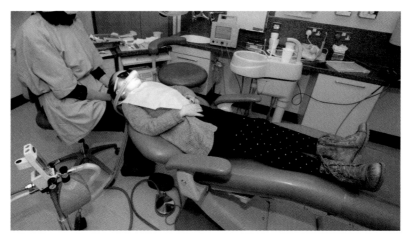

Figure 7.1 A view of surgery, sedated child and essential equipment used for inhalation sedation. Active scavenging is essential and pulse oximeter should preferably be used for monitoring. © M Duggal.

Box 7.1 Essential emergency drugs that should be available

Oxygen
Epinephrine hydrochloride 1:1000 in 1 ml ampoule for IM injection
Hydrocortisone sodium phosphate 100 mg/ampoule
Suitable delivery systems such as needles and syringes
Flumazenil, for reversing oversedation induced by midazolam

Box 7.2 Emergency equipment that should be available for sedation

Positive pressure ventilation with self-inflating bag
Emergency supply of oxygen in addition to working supply
Appropriate face masks for children and adolescents
Various sizes of oral airway
Good high-volume suction with a long extension capacity

Box 7.3 Signs and symptoms of oversedation

Persistent mouth closing
Spontaneous mouth breathing
Patient complains of unpleasant feelings
Lack of cooperation
Nausea and vomiting

Paediatric Dentistry at a Glance, First Edition. Monty Duggal, Angus Cameron and Jack Toumba. © 2013 John Wiley & Sons Ltd. Published 2013 by Blackwell Publishing Ltd.

Definition

Conscious sedation is a technique in which the use of a drug or drugs produce a state of depression of the central nervous system enabling treatment to be carried out, but during which verbal contact with the patient is maintained throughout the period of sedation. The drugs and technique used to provide conscious sedation for dental treatment should carry a margin of safety wide enough to render loss of consciousness unlikely. The level of sedation must be such that the patient remains conscious, retains protective reflexes, and is able to understand and to respond to verbal commands.

Indications

• Children/adolescents who are anxious but potentially cooperative.
• To supplement LA for:
  ◦ potentially traumatic and long procedures, such as multiple extractions and minor surgery;
  ◦ where LA alone is not proving to be effective, such as the extirpation of hypersensitive pulps.
• Children who have an anxiety-related pronounced gag reflex.
• To induce a state of relaxation for systematic desensitisation in children with needle phobia.

Preparing for sedation

An acronym used in the American Academy of Paediatric Dentistry Guidelines (2006) is SOAPME:

S = suction
O = oxygen devices to allow its delivery
A = airway
P = pharmacy: emergency drugs and antagonists like flumazenil (Box 7.1)
M = monitors: pulse
E = special equipment or drugs for a particular case or type of sedation. For intravenous sedation more extensive as indicated (Box 7.2)

Documentation

It is important to keep detailed documentation and records. These should be done:
• before treatment, for consent and preoperative instructions;
• during treatment, for monitoring;
• after treatment, for postoperative recovery period.

Inhalation sedation

This is the most commonly used form of sedation in paediatric dentistry. A mixture of low concentration of nitrous oxide and oxygen is used and the level of nitrous oxide does not usually exceed 50%.

Four key steps are:
• explanation of the procedure using tell–show–do and reassurance;
• administration of the nitrous oxide–oxygen mixture using a titration technique;
• behaviour management with positive reinforcement, and continuous reassurance throughout the procedure;
• effective monitoring by fully trained operator and assistant.

Titration technique

1. Setting the machine to administer 100% oxygen, first set the amount of gas the patient will inhale per minute, usually 2–6 l/min.
2. Once the child is comfortable gradually increase amount of nitrous oxide in increments of 10% until a state of relaxation is achieved.

Signs and symptoms of adequate sedation

What the operator sees (Fig. 7.1):
• patient awake, relaxed and comfortable;
• vital signs, such as pulse rate, within normal limits;
• responds to verbal instruction, such as "open your mouth";
• normal laryngeal reflex but reduced gag reflex;
• decreased response to painful stimuli;
• sluggish response to instruction.

What the patient feels:
• relaxed;
• tingling sensation in extremities;
• euphoric, giggly, warm and comfortable;
• lethargic and dreamy;
• mildly intoxicated and detached.

Scavenging

Due to concerns about repeated exposure to nitrous oxide for staff it is essential to have equipment where scavenging of the exhaled gas is possible with the nasal hood in place. The use of rubber dam for restorative procedures under inhalation sedation is highly recommended as it improves patient comfort and reduces environmental pollution of the surgery with nitrous oxide as it limits mouth breathing.

Oral sedation

Benzodiazepines, and in particular midazolam (0.5–0.7 mg/kg), are most commonly used for oral sedation.
• Most commonly used in pre-cooperative children who will not accept a nasal hood for inhalation sedation.
• Used for short procedure, such as single tooth extraction or short restorative procedure.
• Both the onset and effect are variable and not as predictable as other forms of sedation.
• Longer postoperative supervised recovery period.
• Not recommended to be used routinely by dentists in practice unless suitably trained.

Intravenous sedation

Most commonly used drug is midazolam (0.07 mg/kg). It has a limited use in a general practice and most commonly used in a hospital setting.
• Usually used in older children/adolescents.
• Dentist should be suitably trained in intravenous access and in the monitoring and reversal of sedation.
• Reversal drug flumazenil should be available at all times.

Monitoring of sedated patients

• The dentist and the dental team should be fully trained in the techniques and monitoring of the sedated patient (Box 7.3).
• Active clinical monitoring of the sedated patient should be performed, and if possible a pulse oximeter should be used. This is essential if IV sedation is being used.
• Verbal contact should be maintained with the patient at all times and patient should continue to respond to verbal instruction.
• Adequate recovery facilities should be available.
• Emergency drugs and equipment should always be available and staff trained in their use.
• Emergency protocols should be in place and staff aware and trained in their implementation

Table 8.1 Medical conditions requiring consideration when planning treatment under GA.

Medical condition	Examples
Cardiac	Congenital heart disease, cardiomyopathies and dysrhythmias
Respiratory	Asthma, croup, cystic fibrosis
Haematological	Haemophilia, Von Willebrands, thrombocytopenia, aplastic anaemia, haemoglobinopathies
Immunocompromised	Primary (e.g. asplenia) and acquired (e.g. HIV, chemotherapy)
Endocrine	Diabetes, hypothyroid, hyperthyroid
Metabolic	Malignant hyperthermia, suxamethonium sensitivity
Gastrointestinal	Reflux, difficulty swallowing or feeding
Neurological	Epilepsy, cerebral palsy
Renal	Renal failure, nephrotic syndrome
Liver	Hepatitis, biliary atresia, alpha-1 antitrypsin deficiency
Neuromuscular	Muscular dystrophy
Syndromes	Down, DiGeorge, Williams
Difficult airways	Pierre Robin, sleep apnoea, obesity, cleft palate, micrognathia
Allergies	Latex, penicillin, elastoplast, EMLA, Ametop

Table 8.2 American Society of Anesthesiologists physical status classification system.

ASA grade	Summary
1	A normal healthy patient, i.e. no significant past or present medical history
2	A patient with mild systemic disease
3	A patient with severe systemic disease
4	A patient with severe systemic disease that is a constant threat to life
5	A moribund patient who is not expected to survive without the operation
6	A declared brain-dead patient whose organs are being removed for donation

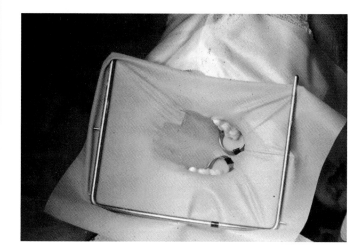

Figure 8.1 The application of rubber dam to isolate both upper and lower arch on the same side under GA, also known as the "double dam" technique.

Paediatric Dentistry at a Glance, First Edition. Monty Duggal, Angus Cameron and Jack Toumba. © 2013 John Wiley & Sons Ltd. Published 2013 by Blackwell Publishing Ltd.

Indications for general anaesthesia

General anaesthesia (GA) carries risks of morbidity and mortality. It should only be considered when treatment using local analgesia or a combination of local analgesia and sedation has failed or is inappropriate. Factors to consider before choosing GA are: the ability of the child to cooperate, the child's degree of anxiety, anticipated surgical trauma, complexity of the procedure (e.g. extractions in multiple quadrants, severe dento-alveolar trauma), presence of acute dental infection, past dental history and medical history of the child (Table 8.1).

Planning treatment under GA

Treatment should be planned with the aim of ensuring all treatment is provided under a single general anaesthetic where possible. Ideally treatment planning should be carried out on a separate day from that of the GA as it allows the parent and child time to consider the proposed treatment. It also gives the dentist the opportunity to liaise with physicians of children who are medically compromised and arrange for preoperative investigations.

The assessing dentist should ideally be a specialist in paediatric dentistry familiar with current evidence and guidelines in the management of the primary and mixed dentition. Radiographs should be obtained where indicated to assist planning. If this is not possible consent should be obtained to take radiographs in theatre. An orthodontic opinion should be obtained if orthodontic extractions are required or when extraction of poor prognosis first permanent molars is required. The need for balancing and compensating extractions should be considered. Consideration should be given to how the medical, dental or social history may influence the treatment plan. In theatre the most predictably successful restoration should be provided. Prevention is an essential component of treatment. It has been shown that failure to adopt a comprehensive approach to planning for GA is highly likely to result in a repeat GA in the future.

Consent

The person obtaining consent should be able to fully explain the procedure, its risks, benefits and alternatives. The operator must satisfy themselves that informed consent has been obtained.

Children 16 years and older can consent for themselves according to the Family Law Reform Act 1969. Those under 16 years can consent for themselves only if deemed to be Gillick competent but it is good practice to involve the parent where possible. Guidelines vary from country to country and it is important for the dentist to be fully conversant with these.

Fasting

Preoperative starvation for children requiring elective surgery aims to reduce the risk of aspiration pneumonia whilst limiting potential problems from thirst, dehydration and hypoglycaemia. Accepted fasting practice is 6 hours for solids and milk, 4 hours for breast milk and 2 hours for clear fluids.

Working with the anaesthetist

Communication is critical. The anaesthetist should be informed of the child's degree of anxiety and whether premedication with a sedative or gaseous induction may be required. Children presenting with upper respiratory tract infections have an increased risk for perioperative complications and should be assessed by the anaesthetist before proceeding with a GA. The anaesthetist should be informed of any known medical factors that may have an influence on the delivery of the general anaesthetic and the recovery of the patient well in advance of the GA (Table 8.1). The American Society of Anesthesiologists (ASA) has devised a simple scale describing fitness to undergo an anaesthetic (Table 8.2). ASA grades 1 and 2 are usually suitable for day stay surgery but grades 3 and 4 require careful preoperative planning in conjunction with the physicians who are looking after them and the anaesthetist. An overnight stay or intensive care bed may be indicated.

Choice of airway

Factors to consider are access required by the dentist, duration of the procedure and medical history of the patient. Choices include:
- **facemask** – suitable for quick simple extractions;
- **laryngeal mask** – compromises access for the dentist but reduces anaesthetic and recovery time;
- **endotracheal tube** – lengthens anaesthetic, improves access;
- **nasotracheal tube** – lengthens anaesthetic, best access, greatest morbidity.

A throat pack of minimal bulk is required to protect the airway without limiting access.

Communication with ward staff

The ward staff may assist in acclimatisation of anxious children by involving play therapists or arrangement of preoperative ward visits. They should be informed of the need for a side room (e.g. cross-infection control, disruptive behaviour, latex allergy).

Choice of analgesia

Analgesic drugs may be administered preoperatively, intraoperatively or postoperatively via the oral, intravenous or rectal route as appropriate. Non-steroidal anti-inflammatory drugs (NSAIDs) and paracetamol are the drugs of choice. NSAIDs alone or in combination with paracetemol provide more effective analgesia than paracetemol alone. Opioids are not routinely required.

Use of local analgesia

Local analgesia in combination with a vasoconstrictor may reduce postoperative bleeding and many anaesthetists prefer its use by the operating dentist.

Use of rubber dam

Rubber dam should be used when providing restorative care. A useful method is to isolate both upper and lower quadrants on the same side together, a technique often called as the "double dam" technique (Fig. 8.1).

Discharge

Verbal and written postoperative instructions should be issued. Analgesics should be recommended for use if indicated. Preventive advice should be reinforced and an appointment for review should be made.

Acknowledgement

The authors would like to kindly thank Sinead McDonnell for her excellent contribution to this chapter.

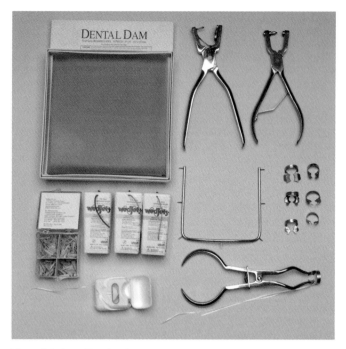

Figure 9.1 The rubber dam kit armamentarium.

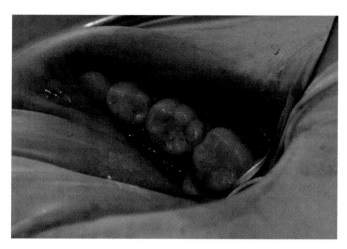

Figure 9.3 Trough technique rubber dam isolation of lower right dental quadrant.

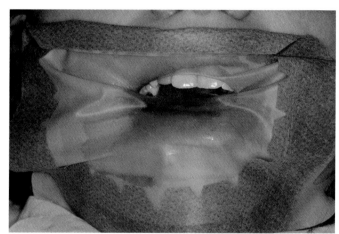

Figure 9.4 Dry dam.

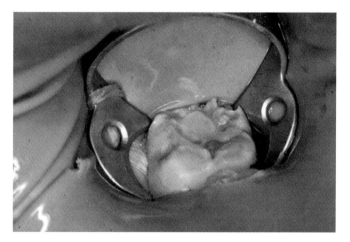

Figure 9.2 Single molar tooth isolation with rubber dam.

Paediatric Dentistry at a Glance, First Edition. Monty Duggal, Angus Cameron and Jack Toumba. © 2013 John Wiley & Sons Ltd. Published 2013 by Blackwell Publishing Ltd.

Background

Rubber dam is usually well tolerated by children as long as they are prepared for its introduction. Once used most patients prefer to have rubber dam during their restorative treatment due to the enhanced intra-oral comfort during the treatment. Rubber dam is quick and easy to apply and with experience takes no more than 1 minute to apply.

History

Rubber dam has been used in dentistry for about 150 years and was first described by Barnum in 1865. UK surveys have shown that less than 2% of dentists routinely use rubber dam.

Indications

- Dental materials requiring moisture control, e.g. composite restorations and fissure sealants.
- Pulpotomy, pulpectomy and all endodontic procedures.

Advantages

- Moisture-free operating field.
- Isolation from salivary contamination.
- Improved access.
- Protection and retraction of soft tissues.
- Improved patient comfort.
- Minimised procedural time.
- Minimised mouth breathing (especially useful when inhalation sedation is being administered).
- Reduced risk of inhalation or ingestion of small instruments or debris (especially during endodontic procedures).
- Cross-infection control is achieved by minimisation of aerosol spread of microorganisms.

Contraindications

- Latex allergy. However, latex-free dam is available and must be used for anyone with a known latex allergy.
- **rubber dam kit equipment:** the rubber dam kit armamentarium (Fig. 9.1) comprises:
- **rubber dam:** latex and latex-free dam of different thicknesses, colours and even tastes are available;
- **rubber dam punch:** the Ainsworth pattern has a wheel with different sized holes whereas the Ash pattern punches a single sized hole;
- **clamps:** a wide range of plain and winged clamps is available but the following six clamps will cover most uses in children:
  - DW – for first and second primary molars;
  - BW – for first permanent molars;
  - K – winged for first permanent molars;
  - FW – a retentive clamp for partially erupted first permanent molars;
  - L – winged for small first primary molars;
  - EW – for primary canines, incisors and premolars.
- **clamp forceps:** Ash, Brewer and Stokes patterns are available;
- **rubber dam frame:** Young's or the modified Young's rubber dam frame are ideal;
- **floss:** a simple loop around the bow is all that is needed to ensure retrieval of the clamp should it become dislodged;

- **additional retention** of the dam can be provided by wooden wedges or latex cord (wedjets).

Technique for rubber dam placement

The technique for placement of rubber dam in children in the primary and mixed dentitions will be described.

Preparation of child for rubber dam

As for all techniques used in paediatric dentistry the child should be prepared by using tell–show–do techniques and using appropriate language for the age of the child. The dam can be described as a "raincoat" and the clamp as a "hat" or "button" whilst the frame can be referred to as a "coat hanger" to keep the coat (dam) straight. Topical and local analgesia are essential to prevent any pain which may ensue if the clamp covers the gingivae. Some individuals like to have a mouth prop for comfort during treatment and prevention of mouth closing which can lead to dislodgement of the clamp.

Single molar isolation (Fig. 9.2)

1. Use a DW clamp.
2. Loop floss over bow of the DW clamp.
3. Punch two overlapping holes in the centre of the dam.
4. Place the clamp onto the tooth at the gingival margin with arch of bow always positioned distally.
5. Ensure the clamp is stable and with floss positioned buccally before removing clamp forceps.
6. Use both index fingers to carry the dam into mouth and stretch the hole to position it over the bow of the clamp.
7. Pull the dam down over the clamp so that the dam is beneath the buccal and lingual aspects of the clamp.
8. Place and secure the frame in place by stretching the dam over the frame prongs.
9. Any excess dam can be folded over and tucked away.

Trough technique for quadrant isolation

This does not provide absolute isolation but is a quick, easy and reliable method which is an excellent method for routine use in children (Fig. 9.3).

1. Clamp the most posterior tooth in the quadrant to be isolated.
2. A row of 5–6 overlapping holes (10–15 mm) is punched in the centre of the dam.
3. The trough is stretched over the clamp as before, hooked over the canine and the frame placed.
4. Additional retention if needed can be provided by wooden wedges or latex cord (wedjets).

Dry dam for anterior teeth

This is ideal for isolating upper incisor teeth. Individual holes or a trough can be punched out for use. There are loops to hook over the patient's ears that hold the dry dam in place and clamps are not normally needed (Fig. 9.4).

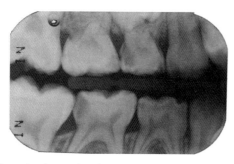

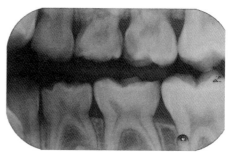

Figure 10.1 Bitewing radiographs showing dental caries.

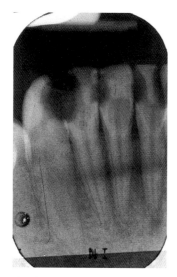

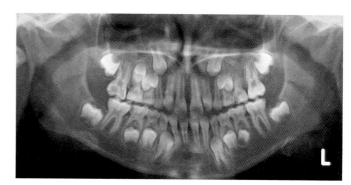

Figure 10.3 Orthopantomogram at developmental stage of child aged 7 years.

Figure 10.2 Periapical radiograph showing dental caries.

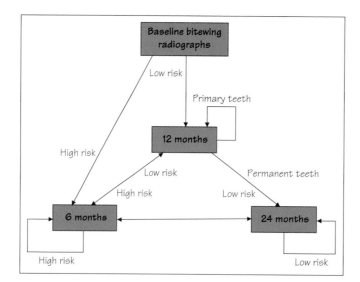

Figure 10.4 Suggested timing of when to take bitewing radiographs in children depending on dental caries risk.

Radiographs in children

Types of radiographs:
- bitewing radiographs (Fig. 10.1);
- periapical radiographs (Fig. 10.2);
- panoramic radiographs (Fig. 10.3);
- lateral oblique radiographs;
- occlusal radiographs;
- computed axial tomography (CAT);
- cone-beam CT with 3D reconstruction.

Radiographic caries diagnosis in children

In a population the use of bitewing radiography in addition to clinical examination increases the number of approximal lesions detected by a factor of between two and eight. The bitewing also offers excellent information about caries in the dentine under occlusal surfaces. During the past two to three decades a number of changes related to bitewing radiography have taken place:
- the decrease in caries prevalence in the western industrialised world – most of these populations experience a skewed caries distribution;
- the relatively slow rate of caries progression in populations regularly exposed to fluoride;
- a revision of the estimates of health detriment caused by exposure to low dose ionising radiation, particularly for children.

Benefits of bitewing radiographs

As an aid for caries diagnosis to:
- detect caries that cannot otherwise be detected;
- estimate the extent of lesions;
- monitor lesion progression.

Good technical quality of the radiographs and good diagnostic quality are essential.

Timing of the first (baseline) bitewing radiographs

When considering the time of the baseline bitewing radiographic examination, adequate selection criteria are necessary including information on:
- relevant epidemiological data on the caries prevalence and rate of progression in the population;
- caries experience;
- oral hygiene and dietary habits;
- exposure to fluorides;
- socioeconomic status.

Based on this knowledge, an individual risk assessment is performed. It should be noted that bitewing radiographs should be taken only if they are considered necessary for adequate treatment.

The primary dentition

Studies in populations with low caries prevalence showed that more than one third of 5-year-olds had approximal carious lesions that could not be detected by visual inspection. In another study between 10 and 60% extra information was gained by the use of bitewing radiographs. Therefore, it seems reasonable to suggest that the 5-year-old should be considered for bitewing examination.

The mixed dentition

At the age of 9 years about one third of a cohort of Swedish children had dentine caries in at least one distal surface of the second primary molar as judged radiographically. Bitewing radiographs at the age of 8–9 years are also useful for deciding the proper interval to the next bitewings.

Minimising ionising radiation exposure

Dental films

D, E and F speed films are available with F speed being the most sensitive.

Digital image receptors

These are usually more sensitive and hence require a significantly lower radiation dose.

Beam collimation

A rectangular collimator offers a significant dose reduction and also results in higher image contrast due to lower scattered radiation.

Extra-oral beam-aiming devices

These reduce misalignment and enable coning of the desired area of interest.

Lead apron protection

A lead apron protects against scattered radiation but has no effect on the gonad dose. If supplemented with a thyroid collar the dose from both primary and scattered radiation to the thyroid gland may be reduced.

Timing of radiographic prescriptions

Fig. 10.4 shows the suggested timing of when to take bitewing radiographs in children depending on dental caries risk. Radiographs form a routine part of dental examinations and it is necessary to repeat radiographs for dental caries diagnosis at appropriate intervals. This will depend on the caries history of the child with 6- and 12-monthly intervals for high and low caries risk children respectively. If a child does not develop new caries lesions at the 6-monthly review then the interval between taking bitewing radiographs can be increased. This interval can progress from 6- to 12- to 18- and 24-monthly intervals but should new or recurrent caries develop at any point the time interval should return to 6-monthly again. At least one orthopantomogram (or its equivalent) should be taken during the developmental stage of the dentition (age 6–8 years).

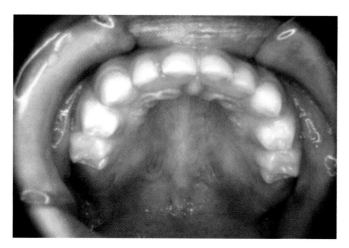

Figure 11.1 Caries-free primary dentition.

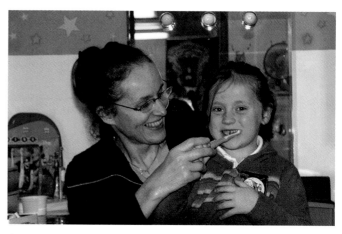

Figure 11.3 Parent and child brushing teeth together. © K J Toumba.

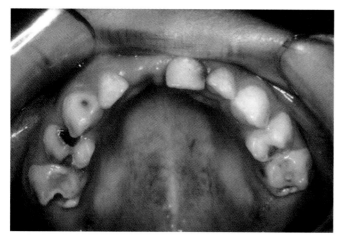

Figure 11.2 Rampant caries in child.

Box 11.1 Dietary advice for prevention of dental caries and dental erosion

Prevention of dental caries
- Do not use sweetened drinks in a bottle or feeder cup
- Discourage prolonged on demand breast feeding (high lactose)
- Recommend safer drinks (water, plain milk and tea) without added sugar
- Recommend safer snacks (fruit, cheese, plain crisps, bread)
- Restrict sugary snacks to mealtimes or one day per week
- Avoid chewy, sticky and boiled sweets
- Be aware of hidden sugars (dried fruits like raisins, yoghurts, flavoured crisps and ketchup)

Prevention of dental erosion
- Avoid acidic foods (citrus fruits, yoghurts, pickled food)
- Limit carbonated and fruit cordial drinks to once a day and preferably at mealtimes
- Use a straw whenever possible
- Do not hold or swish erosive drinks in the mouth
- After an erosive challenge rinse with water or with an anti-erosive rinse
- Eating cheese can raise the oral pH and limit the erosive attack
- Sugar-free chewing gums can help to stimulate salivary flow and buffer oral acidity
- Do not brush teeth after erosive challenges for at least 30 minutes

Pillars of prevention

Dental caries is a preventable disease. The four "pillars of prevention" are:

- plaque control;
- diet;
- fluoride;
- fissure sealants.

Each of these pillars should be incorporated in every preventive treatment plan with the goal of preventing gingivitis, periodontal disease, dental caries and dental erosion. The effects of each of these pillars are additive and the age, cooperation, caries risk and fluoride exposure needs to be taken into account when treatment planning. Prevention should start early and parents should be encouraged to bring their children to the dentist by the age of 6 months so that appropriate oral care advice can be given before any issues arise. Prevention is the foundation of all treatment plans and needs to be individualised for each patient. All treatment plans should start with prevention at the first visit, continue and be reinforced as the course of treatment continues. Applying preventive measures at the start of a course of treatment also fits in with behaviour management strategies for children. Future cooperation and motivation of the child and parent can also be improved by making prevention fun.

Caries risk

This can be classified in a number of ways. A popular method is to classify individuals as low (dmfs = 0 or 1), moderate (dmfs = 2–4) or high caries risk (dmfs ≥5). A simpler method is to use caries-free for those without dental caries and caries-prone for anyone with caries. The decline in caries is bimodal and for young children 75–80% of dental caries occurs in as little as 20–25% of the population (Figs. 11.1 and 11.2).

Parental responsibility

Despite repeated episodes of preventive advice given by the dental team to children and parents the preventive message does not appear to get through to some groups or may be complicated by associated factors such as:

- social well-being;
- medical conditions;
- physical disability;
- psychological impairment;
- developmental delay;
- low socioeconomic groups;
- ethnicity.

This is due to poor patient and parental compliance to follow our guidance and instructions. At the end of the day parents must take responsibility for supervising their child's oral care on a daily basis.

Plaque control

This can be achieved by:

- tooth brushing with a fluoridated toothpaste;
- flossing (with care in older motivated children);
- chemical control with chlorhexidine in selected cases;
- monitoring with plaque disclosure and charting.

Tooth brushing

Parents should be encouraged to start brushing their children's teeth as soon as they start to erupt usually at about 6 months of age. They should use a small soft bristle brush with a smear of toothpaste. The method employed is not important at this stage but parents should be instructed to brush all surfaces of all teeth in order and to also gently brush the gums. As the child grows the parents should supervise their child brushing their own teeth and then to finish off with them brushing the posterior teeth (Fig. 11.3). Children do not develop the manual dexterity to brush their own teeth effectively until they are about 6–7 years old, i.e. when they can tie their own shoe laces. Parents should be advised that it is better to brush their children's teeth whilst standing behind them and with their child's head slightly tilted in a backwards direction which improves visibility and accessibility.

Diet control

Social and behavioural changes are very difficult to achieve and this is the case with dietary modifications. The dietary advice given should be simple, realistic and achievable. Avoid statements like remove all sugars and sweets from your diet. Emphasis should be made to reduce the amount and frequency of intake of sugars and fermentable carbohydrates. The "5 & 2" message is where five meals/snacks (three meals and two snacks) can safely be eaten without causing enamel demineralisation as long as teeth are brushed twice daily for two minutes on each occasion with a fluoride toothpaste containing at least 1000 ppm F. Diet diaries and analysis are of limited value where compliance is poor but are useful in selected cases to highlight cariogenic (or erosive) components, to advise on reducing the amount and frequency of sugar intake and to suggest safer alternatives. Parents should be advised that only water and plain milk should be added to bottles or feeding cups to prevent early childhood caries. Dietary advice for the prevention of dental caries and erosion is shown in Box 11.1.

Fissure sealants

Fissure sealants have been shown to reduce pit and fissure caries of permanent molars by 45–70% in children. There are filled and unfilled sealant types which can be either opaque or tinted. Glass–ionomer cements can be used as interim sealants in patients with poor compliance or in molars that are only partially erupted. They are relatively simple to apply when good isolation and moisture control is achieved. They should be applied as soon as possible after eruption of teeth for caries-prone children and subsequently carefully monitored for leakage. Fissure sealants are indicated for the following priority groups of children:

- caries in the primary dentition;
- siblings with past history of caries;
- caries in first permanent molars;
- continued poor oral hygiene;
- medically compromised;
- special needs and/or learning disability;
- teeth with deep pits and fissures.

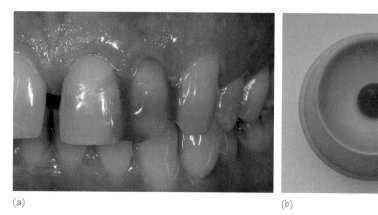

(a)   (b)

Figure 12.1 (a) Excess fluoride varnish application and (b) pea-size amount sufficient for full mouth application in a 5-year-old child.

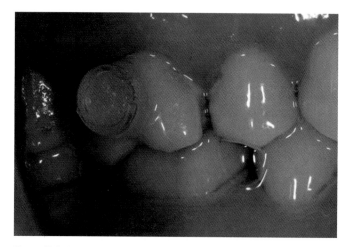

Figure 12.2 Fluoride glass slow-release device attached to maxillary permanent molar.

Table 12.1 Suggestions for fluoride use in some different clinical situations.

Caries 0–6 years	**Caries 6+ years**
F toothpaste (1000+ ppm F)	F toothpaste (1000+ ppm F)
F supplements (0.5 mg/day)	F supplements (0.5 mg/day)
F varnish every 6 months	APF gels or F varnish every 6 months
	Fluoride daily rinse
Rampant caries 0–6 years	**Rampant caries 6+ years**
F toothpaste (1000+ ppm F)	F toothpaste (1000+ ppm F)
F supplements (0.5 mg/day)	F supplements (0.5 mg/day)
F varnish every 3 months	APF gels or F varnish every 3 months
	Fluoride daily rinse
Caries free 0–6 years	**Caries free 6+ years**
Low fluoride toothpaste (<750 ppm F)	F toothpaste (1000+ ppm F)
	Fluoride daily rinse
Orthodontic cases	**Erosion cases**
F toothpaste (1000+ ppm F)	F toothpaste (1000+ ppm F)
Daily fluoride rinse	F varnish
	Daily fluoride rinse

Paediatric Dentistry at a Glance, First Edition. Monty Duggal, Angus Cameron and Jack Toumba. © 2013 John Wiley & Sons Ltd. Published 2013 by Blackwell Publishing Ltd.

Mechanisms of action of fluoride

Tooth tissue mineral exists as a carbonated apatite containing calcium, phosphate and hydroxyl ions, making it a hydroxyapatite [$Ca_{10}.(PO_4)_6.(OH)_2$]. When the pH is below the critical pH for hydroxyapatite (<5.5), demineralisation occurs and when the pH returns to 7.0, remineralisation occurs. Thus there is an equilibrium between demineralisation and remineralisation. When fluoride is present during remineralisation, it forms fluorapatite [$Ca_{10}.(PO_4)_6.F_2$], which is more stable and resistant to further acid attacks. The proposed mechanisms of action for fluoride are:

- it has an effect during tooth formation making the enamel crystals larger and more stable;
- it inhibits plaque bacteria by blocking the enzyme enolase during glycolysis;
- it inhibits demineralisation when in solution;
- it enhances remineralisation by forming fluorapatite;
- it affects the crown morphology making the pits and fissures shallower and hence less likely to create stagnation areas.

It is the activity of the fluoride ion in the oral fluid that is important in reducing the solubility of the enamel rather than having a high content of fluoride in enamel. Therefore a constant supply of low levels of intra-oral fluoride, particularly at the saliva/plaque/enamel interface, is of most benefit in preventing dental caries.

Fluoride formulations

- Sodium fluoride (NaF).
- Sodium monofluorophosphate (NaMFP).
- Stannous fluoride (SnF).
- Amine fluoride (AmF).

Fluoride gels, rinses and varnishes

Topical fluorides should be used in children assessed as being at increased risk for caries development, including children with special oral health care needs.

Fluoride gels

These can be applied in trays or by brush with 26% caries reductions reported. They are high in fluoride (1.23% = 12 300 ppm) for professional use and lower (1000 ppm) for home use. There is a risk of toxicity with the high fluoride containing gels and the following safety recommendations should be followed:

- no more than 2 ml per tray;
- sit patient upright with head inclined forward;
- use a saliva ejector;
- instruct the patient to spit out for 30 seconds after the procedure;
- do not use for children under 6 years of age.

Clinical characteristics

- Long contact time.
- High fluoride concentrations.
- Long intervals between applications.
- Professional application and prescription from a dentist required.

Fluoride rinses

These can be either daily rinses containing 0.05% (225 ppm) or weekly rinses 0.20% (900 ppm) of sodium fluoride. Advise patients to use their fluoride rinses at a different time to tooth brushing so that the number of fluoride exposures increases. Caries reductions of 20–50% have been reported. The effect of tooth brushing and rinsing with fluoride has been shown to be additive. Orthodontic patients should use a daily fluoride rinse to reduce the risk of demineralisation and white spot lesions. Children under the age of 6 years should not be recommended to use fluoride mouth rinses due to the increased risk of swallowing the product.

Clinical characteristics

- Shorter contact time.
- Low fluoride concentrations.
- Short intervals between application.
- Can be implemented by auxiliary dental or non-dental personnel in non-clinical settings.

Fluoride varnishes

Usually are 5% by weight as sodium fluoride = 22 600 ppm F with 50–70% caries reductions reported. It is supplied in a small tube, but used by most as if it were toothpaste. There is the possibility of toxicity with young children. It should be used sparingly (Fig. 12.1) with a cotton bud, a small pea-size amount is sufficient for a full mouth application in children up to 6 years.

Clinical characteristics

- Long contact time.
- High fluoride concentrations.
- Applied in a clinical setting, and can be applied by auxiliary dental personnel.

Each individual patient will require a "tailor-made" fluoride regime, and the dentist will need to use his expertise and knowledge of each patient in formulating individual fluoride regimes and preventive treatment plans. Table 12.1 gives some suggestions for some different clinical situations.

Fluoride glass slow-release devices

The fluoride glass slow-release devices (Fig. 12.2) were developed at Leeds. Studies demonstrated that there were 67% fewer new carious teeth and 76% fewer new carious surfaces in high caries-risk children after 2 years in a randomised controlled clinical caries trial for children with the fluoride devices in comparison to the control group with placebo devices. The fluoride glass devices release low levels of fluoride for up to 2 years and have great potential for use in preventing dental caries in high "caries-risk" groups and irregular dental attenders. The fluoride glass devices have been patented and commercial development in the USA is now under progress.

Table 13.1 EAPD statements for tooth brushing with fluoride toothpaste with level of evidence according to the Scottish Intercollegiate Guidelines Network (2008). Reproduced with permission from Eur Arch Paediatr Dent 2009; 10: 129–135.

Statement SIGN	Level of evidence
Brushing with fluoride toothpaste daily prevents caries	1++
Increasing the frequency of brushing with fluoride toothpaste improves caries prevention	1+
Adult assistance/supervision of tooth brushing in children improves caries prevention	2+
Toothpastes containing higher concentrations of fluoride are more effective than those with lower levels of fluoride in preventing caries	1++
Commencement of tooth brushing prior to 1 year of age reduces the probability of developing caries	3
Ingestion of fluoridated toothpaste by young children is associated with an increased risk of dental fluorosis	2–

Table 13.2 EAPD recommended use of fluoridated toothpaste in children. Reproduced with permission from Eur Arch Paediatr Dent 2009; 10: 129–135.

Age group	Fluoride concentration (ppm)	Daily use	Amount to be used daily
6 months – <2 years	500	Twice	Pea-size
2– <6 years	1000+	Twice	Pea-size
6 years and over	1450	Twice	1–2 cm

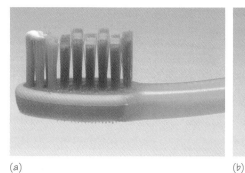

(a)

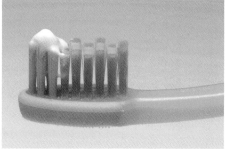

(b)

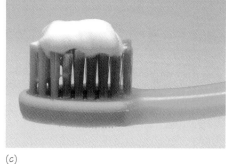

(c)

Figure 13.1 (a) A smear-size amount of toothpaste; (b) a pea-size amount of toothpaste; (c) the full length of brush head amount of toothpaste.

Paediatric Dentistry at a Glance, First Edition. Monty Duggal, Angus Cameron and Jack Toumba. © 2013 John Wiley & Sons Ltd. Published 2013 by Blackwell Publishing Ltd.

Toothpastes

Dental caries levels were observed to decrease worldwide since the introduction of fluoridated toothpastes in the early 1970s.

Toothpaste ingredients

- Abrasives (20–50%): calcium phosphate, calcium carbonate, alumina or hydrated silica (to remove food debris, plaque and to scour off biofilm).
- Water (20–40%).
- Humectants (20–35%): sorbitol and/or glycerol to reduce loss of moisture and to ensure it becomes a manageable paste.
- Surfactants (0.5–2.0%): sodium lauryl sulphate to provide foaming and detergent properties.
- Flavouring and sweeteners (0–2.0%): usually mint to give a pleasant taste.
- Active ingredients (0–2.0%): therapeutic agents such as fluoride, triclosan, potassium nitrate and potassium citrate.
- Gels and binding agents (0.5–2.0%): carboxymethyl and hydroxyethyl cellulose to control the consistency of the paste.
- Colouring and preservatives (0–0.5%).

Toothpaste formulations

These exist as sodium fluoride (NaF), sodium monofluorophosphate (NaMFP), stannous fluoride (SnF) and amine fluoride (AmF). The ionic concentrations of fluoride in dentifrices with different fluoride agents are:

Fluoride agent	500 ppm F	1000 ppm F	1500 ppm F
NaF	0.11%	0.22%	0.33%
NaMFP	0.38%	0.76%	1.14%
SnF	0.22%	0.45%	0.67%
AmF	0.33%	0.66%	0.99%

Levels of fluoride in toothpastes

The most common adult formulations contain 1000 ppm F although the EU directive allows up to 1500 ppm F for over-the-counter sales of dentifrices. Low-fluoride toothpastes containing 500–750 ppm F (and less) are available for children and were introduced to avoid the risk of fluorosis and due to the decreasing caries levels that were being observed. The evidence for the caries preventive efficacy of these low-fluoride pastes is very weak and therefore should not be recommended for caries-risk children. They should be recommended for caries-free children under the age of 6 years especially if they are residing in a water fluoridated area to avoid the risk of ingestion of toothpaste and hence dental fluorosis. Prescription only fluoride toothpastes containing 2800 ppm F and 5000 ppm F are available for high caries-risk individuals.

Dose response of fluoride concentration

For each 500 ppm F increase in fluoride concentration in toothpastes there is a further reduction in caries levels. The additional use of fluoride alongside fluoridated toothpaste has been shown to lead to additional caries reductions. For young children the benefits of caries reduction must be considered alongside the risk of dental fluorosis when increasing the concentration of fluoride in toothpastes.

Brushing behaviours

When to start brushing?

There is evidence (Table 13.1) that caries levels are lower when tooth brushing with a fluoride paste commences before 1 year of age. It is recommended to start brushing children's teeth as soon as they erupt.

Supervision of tooth brushing

Supervised brushing of children's teeth results in lower caries levels than unsupervised brushing (Table 13.1).

Post-brushing rinsing

It is recommended to swish the toothpaste saliva slurry around the mouth to enhance fluoride contact with the teeth and then not to rinse with water but to spit out the excess slurry in order to maintain salivary fluoride levels for as long as possible.

Frequency of brushing

Caries levels are lower (Table 13.1) when tooth brushing frequency is twice a day in comparison to once daily. Ideally tooth brushing should take place first thing in the morning and last thing at night just before bedtime.

Timing of tooth brushing

Ideally tooth brushing with fluoridated toothpastes should occur first thing in the morning before breakfast. Fluoride will be provided just before the acidogenic challenge which will thus limit the amount of tooth mineral loss. Brushing immediately after having breakfast will be when the enamel is softened and further mineral loss will occur due to the abrasion of tooth brushing. If tooth brushing is required after eating this should be after a minimum period of 30 minutes to allow salivary buffering and re-hardening of dental enamel. A good tip is to recommend tooth brushing before breakfast and to use a fluoride dental rinse after breakfast.

Amount of paste to be used

The dose is a product of the concentration of fluoride in the toothpaste and the amount of paste used. For children under 6 years of age it is recommended to use a smear, half-pea or pea size amount of paste rather than the full length of the brush head to minimise the ingestion of fluoride and hence reduce the risk of dental fluorosis (Table 13.2 and Fig. 13.1). The best balance between risk and efficacy might be achieved by using small amounts of high-fluoride toothpaste under close supervision from parents.

Guidelines for fluoride use

There are a number of guidelines that can be referred to in order to help both dentists and patients:
- European Academy Paediatric Dentistry (www.eapd.eu);
- American Academy Paediatric Dentistry (www.aapd.org);
- British Society Paediatric Dentistry (www.bspd.co.uk);
- Department of Health Prevention Toolkit (www.dh.gov.uk).

It should be remembered that these are guidelines and are not mandatory regulations. As such these guidelines should be used to help and guide.

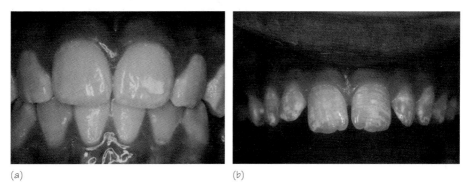

Figure 14.1 Chronic dental fluorosis: (a) demarcated defects of enamel; (b) diffuse defects of enamel.

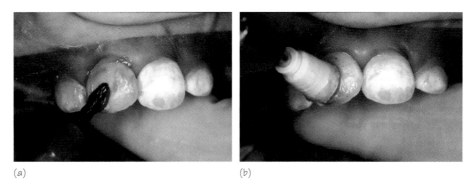

Figure 14.2 Microabrasion technique: (a) isolation of teeth with dry dam and application of acid etchant; (b) abrasion of surface of tooth enamel with pumice.

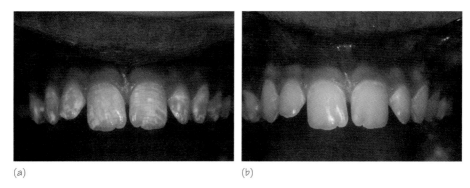

Figure 14.3 (a) Pre- and (b) post-microabrasion of dental fluorosis of upper permanent incisors showing a marked aesthetic improvement.

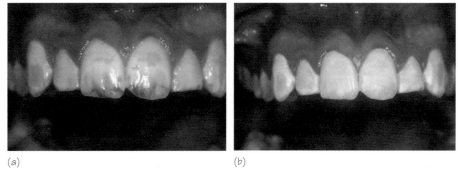

Figure 14.4 (a) Pre- and (b) post-microabrasion of dental fluorosis of upper permanent incisors showing a marked aesthetic improvement.

Systemic fluoridation

- Water fluoridation.
- Fluoride tablets and drops.
- Fluoridated milk.
- Fluoridated salt.

Water fluoridation

Water fluoridation is the controlled adjustment of the natural fluoride concentration in drinking water to that recommended for optimal dental health. The optimum level of fluoride in drinking water was determined as 1 mg/l (1 ppm) from the original 21 cities study of Dean in 1942. Water fluoridation is effective at reducing caries by about 50% (York Review) and has been hailed as one of the 10 greatest achievements in public health in the twentieth century. It is socially equitable, in that it is available to all social groups and ages. With the exception of dental fluorosis, no association between adverse effects and water fluoridation has been established. The development of dental fluorosis is influenced by the total fluoride ingestion from all sources, including toothpaste, during tooth development. Approximately 300 million people drink fluoridated water worldwide. It is not more widespread due to political issues and the anti-fluoride lobby. Cessation of water fluoridation has been shown to lead to increased caries to pre-fluoridation levels within 5 years. In recent years, the use of bottled drinking waters has become more extensive and their fluoride levels may play a role in caries prevention.

Fluoride tablets and drops

Fluoride tablets and fluoride drops (traditionally termed fluoride supplements) were intended to mimic the consumption of fluoride from naturally fluoridated water. Now the common view is that it is through the topical effect on tooth surfaces that fluorides have a caries preventive action and the term "supplements" should be avoided. As the systemic effect of fluoride plays a more minor role in caries inhibition it may be argued that fluorides should be applied locally and not given systemically. The dosage of fluoride tablets and drops varies worldwide and the major drawback of their use is the very poor patient compliance. This explains the wide variation in reported caries reductions with supervised studies having the greatest caries reductions. When used the maximum dose should be 0.5 mg daily and patients should be advised to allow the tablets to dissolve slowly whilst moving the tablet around the mouth so that all teeth benefit from the topical effect of the fluoride release. Recommended dosage schedule (when <0.3 mg F/l in drinking water) is:

- 0–24 months: none;
- 2–6 years: 0.25 mg F/day;
- 7–18 years: 0.50 mg F/day.

They are not to be recommended in areas with water fluoridation. Pre-natal use of fluoride tablets has not been shown to lead to caries reductions and hence is of no benefit. Their use has been linked to increased risk of dental fluorosis.

Fluoridated milk

There is evidence for the caries preventive effect of milk fluoride use in schools and kindergartens. The fluoride concentration in milk is usually in the range 2.5–5.0 mg F/l.

Salt fluoridation

This is widely used in Germany, France and Switzerland with 30–80% of the marketed salt for domestic use being fluoridated More than 30 other countries worldwide use fluoridated salt and this type of fluoride delivery is highly recommended by the World Health Organization. Salt is most commonly fluoridated at 250 mg of fluoride per kg.

Fluoride toxicity

Definitions

Probably toxic dose: 5 mg F/kg body wt.
Safely tolerated dose: 8–16 mg F/kg body wt.
Certainly lethal dose: 32–64 mg F/kg body wt.

- For optimal dental health the total daily intake of fluoride should be 0.05–0.07 mg F/kg body wt.
- To avoid the risk of dental fluorosis intake should not exceed a daily level of 0.10 mg F/kg body wt.
- For permanent central incisors the period of maximum risk is a 4-month period from 22–26 months of age.

Acute fluoride toxicity

Early symptoms:

- nausea;
- hypersalivation;
- vomiting;
- abdominal pain;
- diarrhoea.

Late symptoms:

- convulsions (fall in plasma Ca^{2+} to <2.54 mmol/l);
- cardiac failure;
- respiratory failure;
- death.

Chronic fluoride toxicity

Dental fluorosis (Fig. 14.1)

- Demarcated opacities.
- Diffuse (confluent, patchy, lines).
- Hypoplastic.
- Combinations.

Skeletal fluorosis

- Can be crippling.
- Fusion of intervertebral discs/ligaments.

Osteoporosis

- Fracture of head of femur (elderly and post-menopausal women).

Treatment of dental fluorosis

- Bleaching.
- Microabrasion technique (see Figs. 14.2–14.4):
  1. dry dam or cotton wool isolation;
  2. apply 37% phosphoric acid etchant;
  3. leave for 2 mins (do not wash off);
  4. pumice each surface for 1 min then rinse and dry;
  5. repeat three times at each visit;
  6. apply clear F solution at end of each visit;
  7. 3 × 3 cycles in total.
- Composite/porcelain veneers.

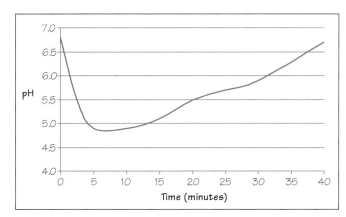

Figure 15.1 A typical Stephan curve showing the plaque pH response to a 10% glucose solution rinse.

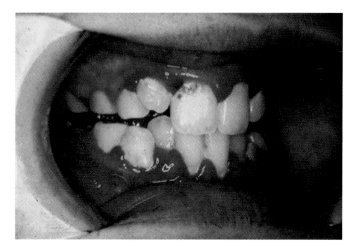

Figure 15.2 Clinical appearance of white spot lesions due to plaque accumulation on buccal surfaces of teeth adjacent to gingival margins.

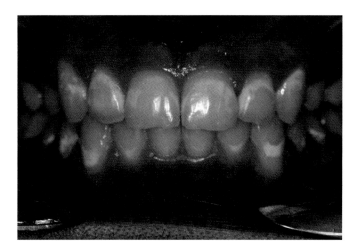

Figure 15.3 Clinical appearance of white spot lesions following orthodontic treatment due to plaque accumulation around the margins of where the brackets were cemented to the buccal surfaces of the teeth.

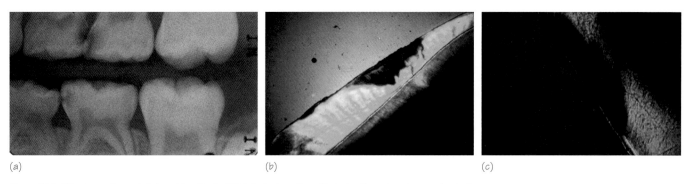

(a)   (b)   (c)

Figure 15.4 Bitewing radiograph (a) and longitudinal histological sections (b,c) showing subsurface caries lesions.

Paediatric Dentistry at a Glance, First Edition. Monty Duggal, Angus Cameron and Jack Toumba. © 2013 John Wiley & Sons Ltd. Published 2013 by Blackwell Publishing Ltd.

Current understanding of cariology

Acidogenic theory

Miller proposed the chemoparasitic theory for the process of dental caries in 1890 which is now commonly known as the acidogenic theory of caries aetiology. The main features of the caries process are:

• fermentation of dietary carbohydrates by microorganisms in plaque to organic acids on the tooth surface;
• rapid lowering of the pH at the enamel surface to below the critical pH (5.5) at which enamel will dissolve;
• following plaque microbial metabolism the pH within plaque will rise due to the outward diffusion of acids and buffering so that remineralisation of enamel occurs;
• demineralisation and remineralisation is an equilibrium so that dental caries progresses only when demineralisation is greater than remineralisation.

Cavitation and subsurface demineralisation

Dental plaque forms on tooth surfaces when tooth brushing is stopped for a few days. Microorganisms comprise 70% of plaque and initially have cocci and then filamentous organisms as the plaque ages. Mutans streptococci are much more numerous when the diet is rich in sugars and fermentable carbohydrates which are metabolised to acids. The early carious lesion of enamel is subsurface with most of the mineral loss beneath a relatively intact enamel surface. The intact surface layer in enamel caries is due to dental plaque acting as a partial barrier to diffusion.

Mechanisms of demineralisation and lesion progression

Robert Stephan researched plaque pH using microelectrodes before, during and after consumption of various foods and drinks. He plotted plaque pH versus time which is now known as a Stephan curve (Fig. 15.1). Within a couple of minutes of rinsing with a 10% sugar solution the plaque pH falls from about 7.0 to near pH 5.0 taking about 30–40 minutes to return to its baseline value. Below pH 5.5 demineralisation of enamel occurs (critical pH).

The clinical appearance of these early lesions is well recognised (Fig. 15.2); they appear as white areas or so-called "white spot lesions" coinciding with the distribution of plaque. White spot lesions are also sometimes seen around orthodontic brackets when oral hygiene is not adequate and plaque has accumulated around the brackets (Fig. 15.3). The subsurface body of the lesion and surface zone are usually seen in radiographs and histological sections of teeth (Fig. 15.4). Progression of caries leads to weakening and breakdown of the surface layer producing a cavity with loss of both enamel and dentine.

Early or "pre-cavitation" carious lesions are able to remineralise. Periods of demineralisation are followed by periods of remineralisation and the balance of this equilibrium determines the outcome between mineral loss and gain. Healing of the carious lesion can only occur if the surface layer is unbroken but once a cavity has formed following surface breakdown a restoration is required.

Diet and dental caries

Daily eating and snacking occasions occur so frequently that it is important to be able to give sensible practical advice regarding diet and dental caries. Many consider that there are "good foods" and "bad foods" whilst others believe that there are "good diets" and "bad diets". Sugar has also been described as the arch villain and enemy of dentistry. However, caries has declined despite increased sales and consumption of sugars. Nevertheless, the literature is controversial and there are many conflicting views and opinions regarding sugar consumption.

Rather than recommending parents to completely stop their children from eating sugary foods we should advise that they eat sensibly and safely. We should advise that only milk or water is given to children in a baby bottle in order to prevent early childhood caries. Young children should be encouraged to consume drinks from trainer cups, beakers and to use straws as soon as possible. "Safer foods" such as cheeses which have been shown to raise plaque pH have been recommended for snacking. Fruit and vegetables, crisps and peanuts have also been recommended as safer alternatives. However, acidic citrus fruits have been implicated in the aetiology of dental erosion and peanuts should be avoided in small children due to possible inhalation risk. The preventive advice is to reduce the frequency and amount of intake of fermentable carbohydrates. The "5 & 2" message is where five meals/snacks (three meals and two snacks) can safely be eaten without causing enamel demineralisation as long as teeth are brushed twice daily for 2 minutes on each occasion with a fluoride toothpaste containing at least 1000 ppm F.

Role of saliva

Saliva is the most important natural defence against dental caries. Dental caries progresses rapidly when salivary flow is impaired. Saliva acts to buffer the pH in saliva and within dental plaque. Saliva is supersaturated with calcium and phosphate which is important in determining the progression or arrest of caries. Fluoride aids the remineralisation process so the intra-oral salivary levels of fluoride are also important.

Functions of saliva

Saliva has many functions as follows:

• ion reservoir – supersaturated with calcium and phosphate ions which promotes remineralisation;
• buffer – neutralises plaque pH after eating to minimise time for demineralisation;
• fluid/lubricant – protects mucosa against mechanical, chemical and thermal irritation;
• cleansing – clears food;
• excretion – secretion of substances;
• antimicrobial – IgA, lysozyme, lactoferrin and sialoperoxidase;
• agglutination – aggregation of bacterial cells;
• pellicle formation – a protective diffusion barrier of salivary proteins formed on enamel;
• taste – acts as a solvent with foodstuff to interact with taste buds;
• digestion – breakdown of starch by salivary amylase.

Box 16.1 The International Caries Detection and Assessment System (ICDAS-II) codes and criteria

Code	Criteria
0	Sound tooth surface: no evidence of caries after prolonged air drying (5 secs)
1	First visual change in enamel: opacity or discoloration (white/brown) is visible at the entrance to the pit or fissure after prolonged air drying
2	Distinct visual change in enamel seen when wet: must be visible after drying
3	Localised enamel breakdown (without clinical visual signs of dentinal involvement) seen when wet and after prolonged air drying
4	Underlying dark shadow from dentine
5	Distinct cavity with visible dentine
6	Extensive (more than half the surface) distinct cavity with visible dentine

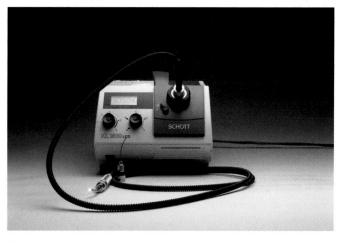

Figure 16.1 The fibre-optic transillumination (FOTI) equipment.

Paediatric Dentistry at a Glance, First Edition. Monty Duggal, Angus Cameron and Jack Toumba. © 2013 John Wiley & Sons Ltd. Published 2013 by Blackwell Publishing Ltd.

Individual caries risk assessment

Caries is a multi-factorial disease with a number of risk factors that can be evaluated to predict caries risk. Practitioners use the demographic, background and social information they collect when taking detailed case histories together with their clinical and radiographic findings and any supplementary tests to come up with a caries risk profile for an individual patient. Determining the caries risk of individual patients will also aid the dentist in planning review appointments and the intervals for subsequent bitewing radiographs. High caries-risk patients are seen at 3-monthly intervals whilst low-risk patients are seen at 6-monthly intervals.

Caries risk assessment factors

Socio-demographic:
- Socio-economic status: low economic levels are associated with high caries risk.
- Educational level: low education levels are associated with high caries risk.
- Ethnicity: first-generation immigrants are at increased caries risk.

Behavioural:
- Diet: high-frequency intakes of cariogenic foods and drinks are associated with high caries risk.
- Fizzy drinks and juices: increased frequency of intake and sipping are associated with high caries risk.
- Habits: swishing and/or holding habits for fizzy drinks and juices are associated with high caries risk.
- Baby bottle: night-time and on demand drinking of cariogenic drinks in a baby bottle are associated with high caries risk.
- Fluoride exposue: irregular or no exposure to daily fluoride is associated with high caries risk.
- Toothbrushing: irregular non-supervised brushing is associated with high caries risk.

Clinical:
- Caries prevalence: past caries is strongly associated with high caries risk.
- Oral hygiene level: plaque index scores >50% are associated with high caries risk.
- Gingival inspection: bleeding on probing is associated with high caries risk.

Radiographic:
- Bitewing radiographs: interproximal as well as new or progression of lesions are associated with high caries risk.

Supplementary tests:
- Salivary flow: low (<0.5 ml/min) salivary flow is associated with high caries risk.
- Salivary buffering capacity: low salivary pH and poor buffering capacity are associated with high caries risk.
- Bacterial: high mutans streptococci or lactobacilli counts are associated with high caries risk.

These caries risk factors are highly variable with only weak evidence for their association with caries risk. By far the strongest predictor of caries risk is previous past risk. Caries risk can be classified in a number of ways. A popular method is to classify young children as low (dmfs = 0 or 1), moderate (dmfs = 2–4) or high caries risk (dmfs ≥5). A simpler method is to use caries-free for those without dental caries and caries-prone for anyone with caries.

Caries detection

Visual inspection

Careful visual inspection of all tooth surfaces is still the best method for detecting dental caries. A number of other systems have been developed to detect dental caries but these must be used with extreme caution as they are prone to both false positives and negatives.

ICDAS-II

The International Caries Detection and Assessment System (ICDAS-II) is a new system for detecting and monitoring lesion progression (Box 16.1) and has been shown to be more accurate than other traditional methods.

Radiographs

Bitewing radiographs detect approximately 40–45% more approximal lesions of molars compared to visual inspection only.

Fibre-optic transillumination (FOTI)

Transillumination of teeth from a buccal or lingual direction aids detection of occlusal lesions. Transillumination from just below the approximal contact point aids detection of interproximal lesions. The different light scattering properties of enamel make it appear as translucent or opaque for sound and demineralised enamel respectively. The fibre-optic transillumination (FOTI) equipment is shown in Fig. 16.1.

Laser light fluorescence

Quantitative light fluorescence (QLF) uses the fluorescent characteristics of teeth and carious lesions. Fluorescent images are quantified and fluorescence loss is directly related to mineral loss and lesion depth using a software package. It is possible to monitor caries lesion de-/remineralisation with QLF.

DIAGNOdent also uses laser fluorescence at a wavelength of 655 nm with the measured red fluorescent light expressed as a number between 0 and 99.

Electronic caries monitor (ECM)

Caries is detected as a fall in electrical resistance due to the porosity of demineralisation.

Tooth separation

The use of orthodontic separators to move teeth apart is very useful for closer inspection of interproximal contact points. Separation usually takes 3–5 days with the teeth returning to their original position within a few hours of removal of the separator.

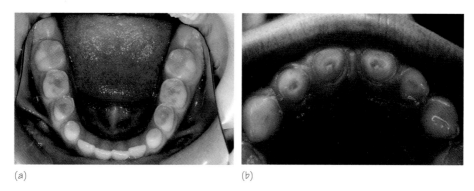

(a)   (b)

Figure 17.1 (a) Dental erosion of lower primary molars. (b) Dental erosion of upper primary incisors.

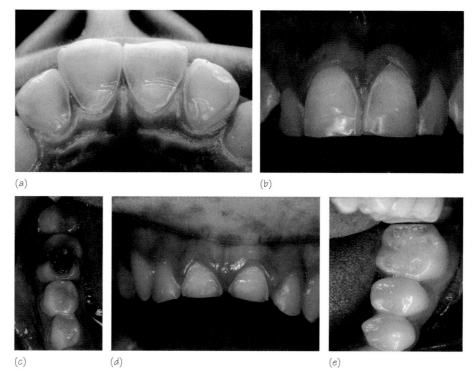

(a)   (b)

(c)   (d)   (e)

Figure 17.2 (a) Palatal enamel surface loss of upper incisors into dentine. (b) Lesions where the breadth exceeds the depth. (c) Edges of restorations standing proud of adjacent tooth surface. (d) Tooth tissue loss disproportionate to age. (e) Cupping of molar cusps.

Paediatric Dentistry at a Glance, First Edition. Monty Duggal, Angus Cameron and Jack Toumba. © 2013 John Wiley & Sons Ltd. Published 2013 by Blackwell Publishing Ltd.

Tooth surface loss

Abrasion, attrition, abfraction and erosion are forms of tooth surface loss that frequently appear together.

• **Abrasion:** loss of tooth structure by mechanical forces from a foreign element.

• **Attrition:** loss of tooth structure by mechanical forces from opposing teeth.

• **Abfraction:** a special form of wedge-shaped defect at the cemento-enamel junction of a tooth as a result of tensile or shear forces provoking micro-fractures or fatigue.

• **Erosion:** the superficial loss of the surface of dental hard tissue by a chemical process which does not involve bacteria (Pindborg).

Prevalence

This varies worldwide from 30–50% (UK), 48% (Ireland), 32% (Germany), 30–35% (Saudi Arabia) to only 5.7% (China).

Pathogenesis

In caries, demineralisation of the crystallites by plaque acid is often followed by remineralisation from saliva. However, erosion is almost irreversible because the organic matrix, on which the hard tissue architecture depends, has also usually been destroyed by overwhelming acid quantities. Both caries and erosion are acid-related diseases with the acid coming from different sources. Bacterial metabolism to produce acid is required for caries but not for erosion. Dietary and behavioural factors are important for both disease processes.

Aetiology

Intrinsic factors

• Gastro-oesophageal reflux disease (GORD): affects 7% of the adult population daily. The most common symptom of GORD is "heartburn".

• Vomiting: either spontaneous or self-induced. It is often associated with an underlying medical condition.

• Rumination (voluntary regurgitation): childhood neglect, abuse and other psychosocial stressors can precipitate rumination in children.

• Bulimia.

• Pregnancy morning sickness.

Extrinsic factors

• Drinks: young age groups tend to drink carbonated beverages, fruit juices and fruit-flavoured mineral waters.

• Foods: particularly citrus fruits, crisps and ketchup. Individual eating habits.

• Medications: many medications induce a dry mouth and some induce nausea and vomiting. In addition some medications are acidic.

Biological (tooth) modifying factors

• Tooth composition and structure.

• Dental anatomy and occlusion.

• Anatomy and configuration of the soft tissues.

• Soft tissue movements.

• Salivary flow rate, composition, buffering capacity and pH.

• Acquired pellicle thickness and diffusive properties of the pellicle.

Chemical (acid) modifying factors

• pH.

• Buffering capacity.

• Total titrateable acidity.

• Type of acid and its dissociation constant (pKa).

• Calcium chelating properties.

• Calcium, phosphate and fluoride ion concentration.

• Physical and chemical properties affecting adherence to enamel and clearance from the oral cavity.

• Ability to stimulate the salivary flow.

• Temperature.

Salivary buffers

• Effective salivary buffering can bring a pH of 3.5 back up to 6.1 in 30 seconds.

• Bicarbonate and phosphate systems.

• Supplementation from the salivary proteins small.

• The relative contribution of each system, and their effectiveness varies with individuals.

• There are various views on defective buffering systems being linked to an increased susceptibility to erosion.

Diagnosis and management

Diagnosis is difficult because of the combinations of wear mechanisms. Dental erosion of primary teeth can progress very rapidly (Fig. 17.1).

Clinical indications of erosion (Fig. 17.2)

• Palatal enamel surface loss of upper incisors into dentine.

• Lesions where the breadth exceeds the depth.

• Wear in areas where there is no tooth-to-tooth contact.

• Edges of restorations standing proud of adjacent tooth surface.

• Tooth tissue loss disproportionate to age.

• Premature exposure of dentine or pulp in isolated teeth.

• Wear more advanced in one arch than the other.

• Cupping of molar cusps.

Practical tips for managing erosive tooth wear

• Dietary/behaviour modification (use of straws and avoidance of swishing habits).

• Assessment of GI status.

• Advice to use soft toothbrush.

• Use toothpastes with high amount of bio-available fluoride.

• Use fluoridated mouthwashes and other products such as remineralising agents at night time.

• Apply fluoride varnish in practice for children at risk of tooth surface loss.

• Alleviation of sensitivity.

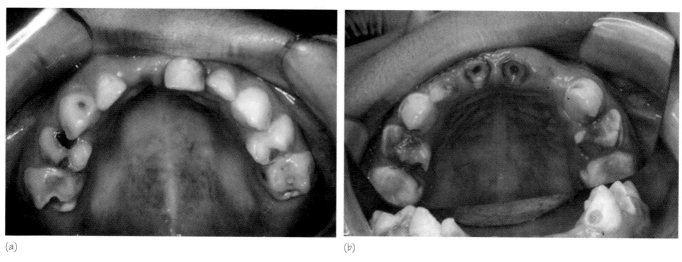

(a)   (b)

Figure 18.1 Early childhood caries (ECC) of maxillary primary incisors and molars.

Box 18.1 Clinical recommendations for the prevention of early childhood caries (from EAPD guidelines based on the Scottish Intercollegiate Guidelines Network (SIGN; www.sign.ac.uk)

- Oral health assessments with counselling at regularly scheduled visits during the first year of life are an important strategy to prevent ECC (grade C)
- Children's teeth should be brushed daily with a smear of fluoride toothpaste as soon as they erupt (grade B)
- Professional applications of fluoride varnish are recommended at least twice yearly in groups or individuals at risk (grade B)
- Parents of infants and toddlers should be encouraged to reduce behaviours that promote the early transmission of mutans streptococci (grade C)
- Frequent intake of sweet drinks and on-demand feeding with sweetened baby bottles should be discouraged, especially at night time (grade C)

Paediatric Dentistry at a Glance, First Edition. Monty Duggal, Angus Cameron and Jack Toumba. © 2013 John Wiley & Sons Ltd. Published 2013 by Blackwell Publishing Ltd.

Early childhood caries (ECC)

The decline in caries is bimodal and for young children 75–80% of dental caries occurs in as little as 20–25% of the population. Allowing young children to sleep with a bottle is one of the main causes of ECC or rampant caries. ECC (Fig. 18.1) occurs worldwide with reported prevalence values ranging from 5% (USA) to 55% (South Korea).

Nomenclature
- Rampant caries.
- Nursing caries syndrome.
- Nursing bottle caries.
- Bottle mouth caries.
- Early childhood caries.
- Severe ECC (S-ECC).

Definitions
ECC: occurrence of any sign of dental caries on any tooth surface during the first 3 years of life.
S-ECC: children with atypical, progressive or rampant patterns of dental caries (described separately for each age group):
- **<3 years:** any sign of dental caries in smooth surfaces;
- **3–5 years:** one or more cavitated, missing (due to caries) or filled smooth surfaces in maxillary teeth or a dmfs score of 4, 5 or 6 surfaces for ages 3, 4 and 5 years respectively.

Aetiology
- Exposure for long periods of time to cariogenic substrates (usually sugary drinks) in nursing bottles and/or feeder cups given as pacifiers.
- Nursing bottle given at bedtime.
- Low salivary rates at night.
- Reduced buffering capacity.
- Parental history of caries (especially mother).
- Associated with low socio-economic status.
- Associated with low educational level of parents.
- Associated with ethnic minorities.
- On-demand breast feeding continued after 1 year of age.

Initiation and progression of ECC
- Prolonged habit of feeding from a nursing bottle combined with poor or usually no oral hygiene measures.
- Decreased salivary flow at bedtime whilst demineralisation process continues.
- Appearance of white spot (demineralisation) lesions on buccal surfaces close to the gingival margins of the maxillary incisor teeth.
- Canines are affected very late on due to their later eruption dates.
- Progression leads to cavitation of the lesions and as the primary molars erupt they develop caries.

- Disto-occlusal cavities in all first primary molars and occlusal cavities in second primary molars.
- Lower primary incisors and canines are usually unaffected due to copious salivary bathing of these teeth from the adjacent sublingual and submandibular salivary glands as well as some protection from the tongue.
- Progression leads to further breakdown, pulpal involvement, loss of vitality and abscess formation.
- At presentation the maxillary incisors are frequently present as stumps and beyond repair.

Management of ECC
Preventive
The clinical recommendations for the prevention of early childhood caries (from EAPD guidelines on ECC, www.eapd.eu) are shown in Box 18.1.
- Explanation of causes without apportioning blame.
- Education and advice to stop the habit.
- Dietary advice.
- Oral hygiene instruction and tooth brushing instruction.
- Fluoride applications.

Restorative
- Assess cooperation of child and decide on whether treatment will be conducted using local analgesia, sedation or general anaesthesia.
- Build-up of restorable anterior teeth with composite resin strip crowns.
- Restoration of primary molars depending on extent of caries and cooperation of child with either composite, glass ionomer cement, pulpotomy, pulpectomy and preformed metal crowns (SSCs).
- Extraction of any unrestorable primary teeth.
- Fissure sealant placement of all first permanent molars on eruption.
- Review and monitor clinically and radiographically at 3–6-monthly intervals and reinforce the intensive preventive regimes started.

Other points
- General anaesthesia is frequently needed to treat young children with ECC.
- Loss of the upper primary incisors does not result in space loss.
- Speech develops normally.
- Loss of primary molars may lead to space loss and a space analysis should be performed to determine whether a space maintainer is needed. This is especially the case for the second primary molars whose early loss can lead to mesial positioning of the first permanent molars.

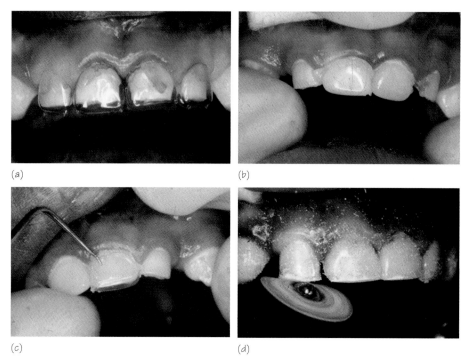

(a)

(b)

(c)

(d)

Figure 19.1 (a) Trimmed strip crowns are try-in fitted to check margins and cervical fit. (From Duggal et al., 2002, with permission.) (b) Strip crown forms containing composite resin are seated on the prepared teeth. (c) The incisal edge of the celluloid strip crown is penetrated and "stripped" off using a probe or an excavator. (d) The crowns are smoothed and polished using Soflex discs or Baker Curson burs. (From Duggal et al., 2002, with permission.)

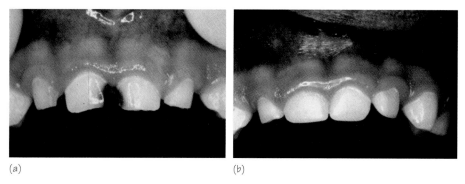

(a)

(b)

Figure 19.2 An example of a case where carious upper central incisors (a) were restored with strip crowns (b).

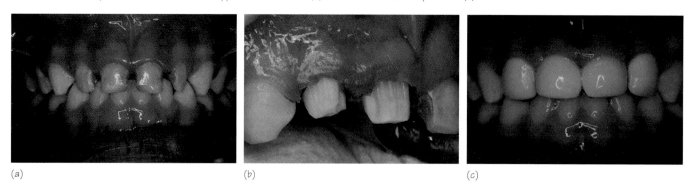

(a)

(b)

(c)

Figure 19.3 Carious upper central incisors (a), prepared (b) and restored with NuSmile crowns (c). Courtesy of Dr Theodore Croll, NuSmile crowns.

Paediatric Dentistry at a Glance, First Edition. Monty Duggal, Angus Cameron and Jack Toumba. © 2013 John Wiley & Sons Ltd. Published 2013 by Blackwell Publishing Ltd.

Introduction

Poor aesthetics of the primary incisors is a common reason for parents bringing their child to the dentist for the very first time. The most common cause of the unsightly appearance of the primary incisors is dental caries as a consequence of early childhood caries with a history of feeding with a nursing bottle. Aesthetic concerns in a young child should not be disregarded. Many dentists are reluctant to offer aesthetic restorations for carious primary incisors. There is no justification for this attitude and all attempts must be made to restore carious primary incisors after the cause of dental caries is diagnosed and eliminated and a preventive regime has been instituted. Some excellent options for restoring carious primary incisors are available ranging from simple composite restorations, use of strip crowns or preformed veneered anterior crowns.

Treatment options

The stage of decay of the primary incisors as well as the age and cooperation of the child will determine the treatment option. A comprehensive preventive programme including dietary advice, oral hygiene instruction and fluoride use is a prerequisite before any restorative treatment can commence. The caries process must be arrested and further caries prevented. One of the treatment options is interproximal disking of the affected incisors to render them self-cleansing (result is usually not aesthetically pleasing). Composite restorations may be sufficient if the caries is confined to a single surface but anything more extensive requires a composite strip crown.

Strip crowns

Indications

- Extensive or multi-surface caries in primary incisors.
- Congenitally malformed primary incisors.
- Congenitally discoloured primary incisors.
- Primary incisors discoloured following trauma.
- Fractured primary incisors.
- Amelogenesis imperfecta.

Technique

See Fig. 19.1.

1. LA and isolation of primary incisors with dry dam.
2. Measure mesio-distal width and select size of celluloid.
3. The shade of composite resin is selected.
4. The celluloid crown is trimmed and vent holes are made in the incisal corners of the crown.
5. Remove all caries with round burs in a slow-speed handpiece.
6. The length of the crown is reduced incisally with a tapered diamond or tungsten carbide bur in a high-speed handpiece.
7. Mesial and distal slices are prepared.
8. The trimmed crowns are trial fitted.
9. Apply Vitremer liner if required.
10. Etch teeth for 20 seconds, wash and air dry.
11. Apply bonding agent and cure.
12. Fill crown form with composite.
13. Hollow out composite to reduce excess.
14. Seat filled crowns on prepared teeth.
15. Remove excess composite with a flat plastic and a probe.
16. Light cure composite crowns for 1 minute labially and palatally.
17. Strip off crown form with probe or Soflex discs.
18. Smooth and polish crowns with disks and finishing burs and check labial and palatal surfaces.

Practical tips

- The end result depends on how accurately the celluloid strip crowns are trimmed. This can be achieved and chair side time also reduced by taking a sectional alginate impression that spans between the upper primary canines at the treatment planning stage. This is of most benefit when strip crowns are indicated for all four upper primary incisors. Each crown can be selected and carefully trimmed before the patient attends.
- When preparing multiple strip crowns place and cure the two central primary incisors first before the lateral incisors.
- When stripping off the celluloid crown formers do so from the palatal surface to avoid damage to the labial surface. Alternatively use a Soflex disc to remove the incisal edge of the crown just into the composite material to allow stripping of the crown former with a probe from the palatal surface.
- Retention can be improved if needed by creating small undercut grooves in the palatal and/or labial surfaces at the preparation stage. This is not normally needed due to the great adhesive properties of modern restorative materials. An example of a treated case is shown in Fig. 19.2.

Pre-veneered crowns – NuSmile^R

These are an alternative to strip crowns and are stainless steel anterior crowns with a aesthetic resin veneer. They are cemented using a glass ionomer cement after the tooth has been adequately prepared. They can be useful when the remaining tooth structure is not considered to be of adequate quality or quantity for a composite restoration to be placed, with or without the use of a strip crown. NuSmile incisor crowns, which are very aesthetic, can be used as an alternative to composite strip crowns. A definite finishing line, which should be subgingival, has to be created which requires an extensive tooth preparation than when strip crowns are used. Children should be given oral hygiene instructions to brush in this region carefully to prevent gingivitis from developing. They also cost more, but are an acceptable alternative in some patients and should be considered (Fig. 19.3).

Review

Both patients and parents are delighted by the vast improvement in the appearance of the teeth that motivation for oral dental health also improves drastically. Oral preventive advice should be reinforced on completion of strip crowns and at subsequent review visits during these enhanced receptive periods. The improved oral health can be supervised and monitored into adulthood.

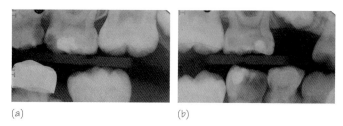

(a)　　　　　　　　　　　(b)

Figure 20.1 Bitewing radiographs showing composite restorations that have failed because of inadequate removal of caries and also poor preventive control following restorations.

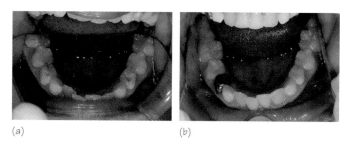

(a)　　　　　　　　　　　(b)

Figure 20.2 Mesial caries in 85 (a) which was considered suitable for restoration with composite restoration (b).

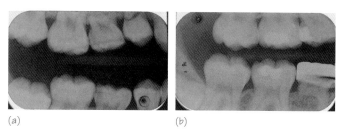

(a)　　　　　　　　　　　(b)

Figure 20.3 Bitewing radiographs showing distal caries in 64 (a) which was not clinically visible and was suitable for restoration with composite resin (b).

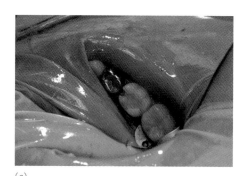

(a)

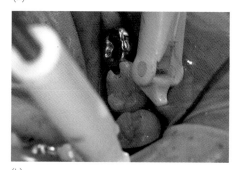

(b)

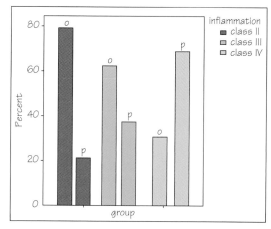

Figure 20.4 Distribution of teeth with caries depth <50% of dentine thickness according to caries site. It can be seen that severe inflammation (class IV) is more likely to be present with proximal caries (P), compared with occlusal caries (O) (Kassa et al, 2008).

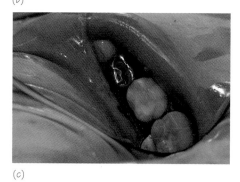

(c)

Figure 20.5 Placement of composite restoration in 85.

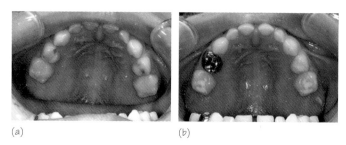

(a)　　　　　　　　　　　(b)

Figure 20.6 Disto-occlusal composite restorations placed in 64. The rest of the susceptible surfaces and teeth were fissure sealed.

Paediatric Dentistry at a Glance, First Edition. Monty Duggal, Angus Cameron and Jack Toumba. © 2013 John Wiley & Sons Ltd. Published 2013 by Blackwell Publishing Ltd.

Introduction

Wedging a dollop of glass ionomer cement between cavity walls after inadequate removal of caries without local analgesia is not good-quality restorative dentistry and it is no surprise that such restorations frequently fail. All efforts should be made to provide good-quality restorative care for carious primary teeth, with restorations that are performed to standards that do not circumvent the basic principles of restorative dentistry. Two important principles are removal of all caries, which is only possible after achieving good pain control with administration of local analgesia, and the prevention of secondary caries (Fig. 20.1). For restorations to be successful and to last for the lifetime of the primary molars the following need to be considered:

• What is the **size and site** of the lesion?
• Is the **pulp healthy or is it likely to be inflamed**?
• Are the **properties of the material** being considered for use compatible with the planned restoration?

Size and site of lesion

Plastic restorations have the best outcome for small lesions affecting one or two surfaces. Full coverage, such as with stainless steel crowns, should be provided for more extensive and multi-surface caries. In the author's opinion plastic restorative materials perform the best for:

• occlusal cavities;
• small proximal caries that involve less than a third of the marginal ridge (Fig. 20.2);
• proximal caries that is not clinically evident but diagnosed on bitewings (Fig. 20.3).

State of the pulp

One of the reasons for failures associated with placing proximal restoration in extensively decayed primary molars is that pulp inflammation sets in early for proximal caries (Chapter 21), and precedes the exposure of the pulp. Also, pulp inflammation seems to be worse for occlusal caries compared with proximal caries. Proximal carious lesions extending to more than 50% through dentine thickness appear to have significantly more extensive inflammatory pulpal changes than teeth with occlusal caries of the same depth (Fig. 20.4). Large restorations placed in such situations often fail.

Properties of materials

Assess whether the size and site of the lesion is compatible with the known properties of the material being used. For example, where there is a large proximal cavity with symptoms of reversible pulpitis, an excellent seal is required to allow the pulp to heal. A composite restoration in such a situation would not be able to provide such a leak-proof seal, and a full coverage would be more suitable. Also isolation and child's behaviour will have an impact on material chosen. Composites are not suitable in cases where isolation is likely to be poor. Glass ionomers are not suitable for restoration of all but the smallest cavities, and also should not be considered for restoration of proximal surfaces.

Amalgam

Amalgam has a long history of use and it is the least technique- and moisture-sensitive material. It works well for occlusal and multi-surface restorations. However, concerns about its environmental and health impacts have led to a steady decline in its use especially in children.

Composite resin

Composite resin is the preferred restorative material for most situations. However, most studies suggest that it does not perform as well in primary molars, especially for proximal restorations. Composite resin restorations must be performed in a dry field (Fig. 20.5) and as most dentists in practice do not routinely use rubber dam for the restoration of primary teeth, this probably accounts for poor outcomes. Also composites are technique and moisture sensitive, undergo polymerisation shrinkage and are susceptible to wear and deterioration due to instability in water.

Indications for use in primary molars are:
• occlusal and small proximal lesions;
• in conjunction with preventive resin restoration (PRR);
• after pulp therapy, if a stainless steel crown is not available or used. In such situations a two-layer restoration, also sometimes called a "sandwich" restoration is carried out, with a base layer of GIC and then composite to complete the restoration.

Glass ionomer cements (GIC)

Despite significant recent improvements in the modern GIC, they have limited indications for restorations of primary molars. Many studies and systematic reviews have shown that they do not perform well in primary molars except when used for restoration of occlusal caries. Multi-surface cavities should not normally be restored with GIC. They are extremely moisture sensitive and need a dry field for placement. An important advantage over composite resins is that GIC do not suffer from polymerisation shrinkage. Also, fluoride release from GIC is considered an advantage.

Indications for use are:
• occlusal lesions of any size;
• as PRR with fissure sealant placed in the rest of the susceptible occlusal surface;
• temporary stabilisation of the extensively carious primary dentition before a full restorative and preventive treatment plan is implemented;
• restoration of caries on the buccal surface;
• as a base layer in multi-layered restorations as it is compatible with composite resins.

Other restorative materials

• Resin-modified GIC.
• Polyacrylic modified composite resins (compomers).

These are widely available and used in similar situations where composite resins would be considered.

When a restoration is placed on any surface of the primary molar, it is good practice to fissure seal the remaining susceptible surfaces at the same time (Fig. 20.6).

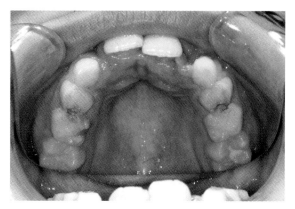

Figure 21.1 Intra-oral photograph showing example of marginal ridge breakdown. The pulp in such cases is usually inflamed and a pulpotomy is required.

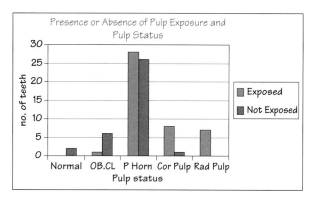

Figure 21.2 Relationship between extent of caries and pulp inflammation. It can be seen that in primary molars where caries has resulted in breakdown of the marginal ridge, even when the pulp is not clinically exposed pulp inflammation is already present in the pulp horn (Duggal et al, 2002).

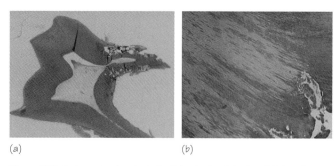

(a)

(b)

Figure 21.3 Caries extending to half of the depth of dentine (a), but the bacteria have already penetrated the tubules through to the pulp (b).

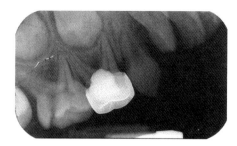

Figure 21.4 Radiograph showing furcation pathology present in upper first primary molar. Infection in primary molars always manifests in the furcation region due to presence of accessory communications between the pulp and furcation region.

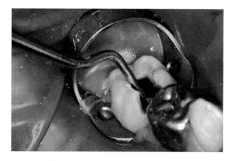

Figure 21.5 Removal of the coronal pulp using sharp excavators.

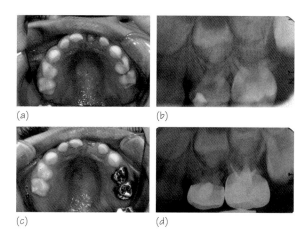

(a)

(b)

(c)

(d)

Figure 21.6 (a,b) Caries in 64 and 65. (c,d) 64 was treated with a pulpotomy and restored with a SSC. Pulpectomy was performed in 65.

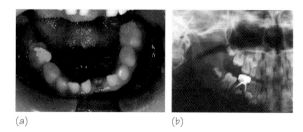

(a)

(b)

Figure 21.7 (a) A patient with an otherwise intact dentition but caries in 85 which resulted in an abscess. (b) This was treated with a pulpectomy.

Paediatric Dentistry at a Glance, First Edition. Monty Duggal, Angus Cameron and Jack Toumba. © 2013 John Wiley & Sons Ltd. Published 2013 by Blackwell Publishing Ltd.

Diagnosis of pulp status

Pulp inflammation sets in early for proximal caries, and precedes the exposure of the pulp. There is evidence that pulp inflammation is already present in cases where proximal caries involves more than half the width of the marginal ridge (Fig. 21.1) or more than half the depth of dentine, even before the pulp is clinically exposed (Fig. 21.2). Bacteria can penetrate the wide dentinal tubules and reach the pulp ahead of the carious lesion and cause pulpal inflammation (Fig. 21.3). Also, history of pain and discomfort is carefully assessed. Pain that makes the child cry, lingers or wakes the child up at night is indicative of irreversible pulpitis.

Direct pulp capping

This is not considered for carious exposures in primary molars. A pulp exposed through the caries process is inflamed as discussed in previous sections.

Indirect pulp capping

See Chapter 23.

Pulpotomy

Pulpotomy involves the removal of coronal pulp which is deemed to be inflamed, thereby leaving the healthy radicular pulp in situ. A restoration that provides an excellent coronal seal to prevent reinfection of the remaining pulp tissue is then placed.

Indications

• Deep proximal caries.
• No history of spontaneous or persistent pain, or evidence of infection, such as furcation radiolucency (Fig. 21.4).
• Instances where extraction might not be desirable, such as in patients with haemophilia and other bleeding disorders.

Contraindications

• In children with congenital heart disease or immunosuppression.

Pulpotomy technique

1. Good analgesia and rubber dam application.
2. Remove caries and roof of the pulp chamber.
3. Remove coronal pulp with excavators or large round bur (Fig. 21.5).
4. Arrest bleeding with dry cotton pledget and then with ferric sulphate applied for 30 seconds to 1 minute.
5. Place a base over pulp. Zinc oxide eugenol (Kalzinol) is commonly used, but mineral trioxide aggregate (MTA) gives a better outcome.
6. A good coronal seal is required. Stainless steel crowns have best outcome, in which case the cavity can be filled with any material, even zinc oxide eugenol. If composite is being used, a layer of glass ionomer is placed first beneath the composite.
7. Regular clinical assessment and normally only occasional radiographic assessment is required, no more than twice over the life time of the tooth (Fig. 21.6).

Pulpotomy medicaments

A pulpotomy is only carried out if the pulp inflammation is suspected to affect the coronal pulp and the radicular pulp is deemed healthy. Therefore, the use of a fixative, such as formocresol, is not indicated and should not be used. There are also concerns regarding its toxicity. In the last decade excellent results have been reported with 15.5% ferric sulphate (Astringident[R]). MTA has also been used successfully but its cost remains prohibitive.

Pulpectomy

This involves gaining access to the root canals, removal of inflamed or infected tissue and filling the root canal with a suitable material that will help preserve the primary tooth in the arch in a non-infected state (Fig. 21.7).

Indications

• Primary molars that have irreversible pulpitis.
• Primary teeth with necrotic pulps.
• Evidence of furcation radiolucency on the radiographs.
• Presence of a chronic or acute abscess where tooth needs to be maintained in the arch.

In many such situations extraction could also be considered as a valid treatment option and a pulpectomy is carried out if the preservation of the primary molar is deemed essential.

Pulpectomy technique

If an acute abscess and/or cellulitis is present then antibiotics need to be administered and drainage established to relieve acute symptoms. Drainage can be established through the carious cavity. Pulpectomy can then be performed when acute symptoms have subsided. The technique is:
1. Good analgesia and rubber dam application.
2. Remove caries, roof of the pulp chamber and identify root canals.
3. Use a barbed broach first to remove any granulation tissue or necrotic material, and irrigate.
4. Lightly clean the root canals with files, copious irrigation and dry with paper points.
5. Fill the root canal with a material which will resorb with the resorbing root such as pure zinc oxide eugenol or Vitapex[R] (contains iodoform and calcium hydroxide). Use files to carry material into root canal or carefully use spiral root fillers.
6. Good coronal seal and preferable full coverage with stainless steel crown.
7. Postoperative radiograph and regular reviews.

Management of acute facial swellings

Antibiotics should only be prescribed in children if a dental abscess is associated with facial swelling and systemic symptoms. Antibiotics are not required for "gum boil" or a draining sinus. Choice of antibiotics is described in Chapter 53. In addition local measures, such as establishing drainage, often through the carious cavity, are required.

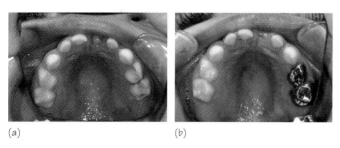

(a)   (b)

Figure 22.1 SSC used to restore multi-surface caries.

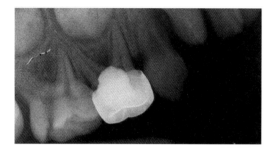

Figure 22.2 SSC used to restore upper first primary molar after pulpotomy.

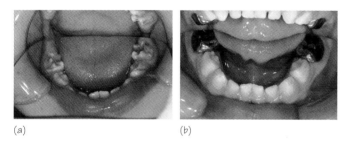

(a)   (b)

Figure 22.3 SSC used to restore hypomineralised primary second molars.

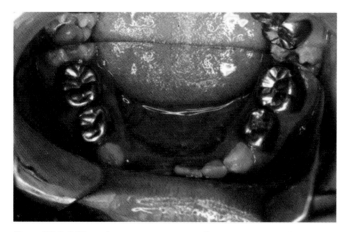

Figure 22.4 SSC used to restore primary molars in a patient with amelogenesis imperfecta.

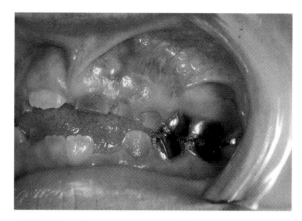

Figure 22.5 SSC used to restore primary molars in a patient with dentinogenesis imperfecta.

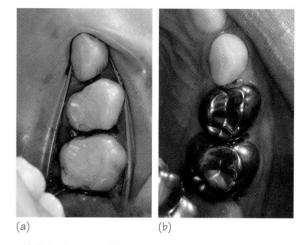

(a)   (b)

Figure 22.6 Tooth prepared for placement of SSC. Note reduction of only proximal and occlusal surfaces (a) before seating the selected crowns (b).

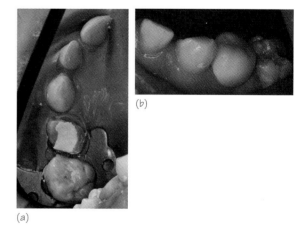

(b)

(a)

Figure 22.7 Aesthetic crowns (NuSmile). Tooth preparation (a) and placement of the NuSmile Crown (b). Courtesy of Dr Karin Ziskind, NuSmile Crowns.

Paediatric Dentistry at a Glance, First Edition. Monty Duggal, Angus Cameron and Jack Toumba. © 2013 John Wiley & Sons Ltd. Published 2013 by Blackwell Publishing Ltd.

Stainless steel crowns (SSC)

This has proved to be the most successful restoration for carious primary teeth. It is long lasting and versatile enough to be used in many situations for the restoration of the primary dentition and also permanent molars in children and adolescents. Stainless steel crowns are supplied only by 3M ESPE.

Indications

• Restoration of primary molars with caries involving multiple surfaces (Fig. 22.1).
• Restoration of primary molars after pulp therapy or after indirect pulp capping (Fig. 22.2).
• Children with rampant caries who will benefit from full coverage.
• Restoration of primary molars with developmental defects. Particularly useful for the protection of the primary dentition in cases of amelogenesis and dentinogenesis imperfecta (Figs. 22.3–22.5).
• Restoration of extensively carious primary molars in pre-schoolers where a truly long lasting restoration is required.
• In children with disabilities with severe bruxism that is causing damage to the dentition. SSCs protect tooth surface wear in these situations and often need to be placed under general anaesthesia.
• Restoration of hypomineralised permanent molars, such as occur in cases of molar incisor hypomineralisation (MIH), see Chapter 25.

Technique (Fig. 22.6)

1. Reduce the occlusal height of the tooth by 2–3 mm or until the tooth is completely out of occlusion.
2. Mesial and distal reduction with the aim being to make clearance for seating of the crown. Care is taken not to damage the adjacent teeth and that no step is created that would stop the seating of the crown.
3. Select a crown for a trial fit. With experience an estimate is easily made of the probable size, but sometimes several have to be tried until one fits. The crown should seat with a "snap". Most crowns seat best if seated lingually first and rotated on to the buccal surface.
4. Crimp the edges slightly.
5. Cement the crown with glass ionomer cement.
6. Remove excess cement and make a final check of the restoration. No buccal or lingual/palatal reduction is required. In the upper first primary molars where some space has been lost due to proximal caries, occasionally a slight palatal reduction may be needed to facilitate crown placement.

A slight discrepancy in the occlusion adjusts within a few days. Also, blanching of the gingival tissues around the margins of the crown should be disregarded as children report little postoperative discomfort after the placement of SSCs.

Advantages

• **Low failure rate.** Once placed SSCs seldom come off. Failure rates of less than 5% over 5 years have been reported.

• **Easy to place.** Once the technique is learnt, it takes less time than preparing and placing a class 2 restoration with composite resin.
• **Cost-effective.** Because of ease of placement and low failure rates it is the most cost-effective restoration.

Repeated replacements of restorations in children has implications for the child's behaviour. In view of the very low failure rates reported with SSCs all clinicians who treat children should be familiar with this technique.

Concerns about aesthetics

In the authors' experience very few parents or patients express concerns about the aesthetics of stainless steel crowns. There will be cultural differences and these may be less acceptable in some countries than others. Sometimes it is possible to cut out the buccal part of the crown after cementation and replace this with a composite at the chair side to improve the aesthetics. Alternatively, aesthetic crowns are commercially available.

Aesthetic crowns for primary molars
Pre-veneered NuSmile^R crowns (Fig. 22.7)

For those who are concerned about aesthetics of the SSC, pre-veneered stainless steel crowns such as NuSmile crowns are available. The technique differs from the traditional SSC preparation and considerably more tooth preparation is required. The tooth should be reduced occlusally and proximally, but also buccally and lingually/palatally. About 30% tooth reduction is required to accommodate the crown and to create subgingival feather-edge margins. A "snap" fit as for SSC is not desirable for these crowns due to the risk of fracture of the resin veneer. Once learnt and with a little practice the technique is easy to use for a specialist paediatric dentist. The aesthetic outcome is excellent and the resin veneer is durable and the crown long lasting if cemented with glass ionomer cement.

The Hall technique

Recently there has been some literature on the use of conventional stainless steel crowns in children but using no or minimal caries removal and no tooth preparation. Without using local analgesia, the crown is seated forcibly with finger pressure, or with the child biting down on the crown. The proponents of this technique claim that this does not cause excessive discomfort for the child and once the crown is cemented caries progression slows or stops due to the nature of the seal, and deprivation of substrate for the bacteria. The technique was designed for use in a very high caries regions of Scotland in young children with multiple caries. There is some literature to support the use of this technique, and due consideration may be given to its use in such situations where little else is possible.

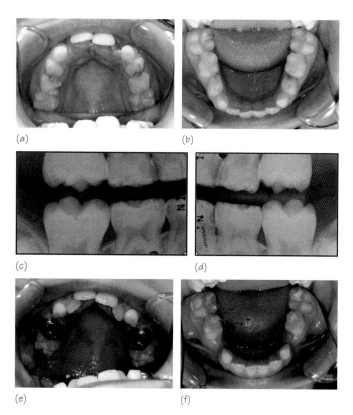

Figure 23.1 Facial cellulitis in a child resulting from an abscess on a poorly restored upper primary molar.

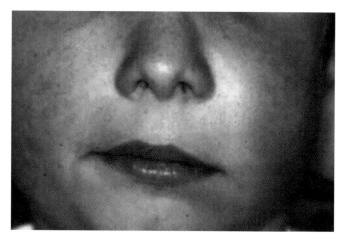

(a)　　　　　　　　　　　(b)

(c)　　　　　　　　　　　(d)

(e)　　　　　　　　　　　(f)

Figure 23.2 An example of a young patient who was very anxious with all primary molars affected with dental caries. It was considered in the child's best interest to restore the second primary molars and extract the first primary molars.

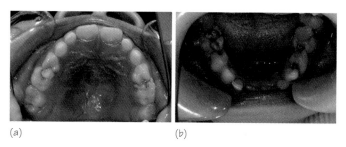

(a)　　　　　　　　　　　(b)

Figure 23.3 ART-type restorations that have failed since placement, resulting in the patient now requiring extensive restorative care.

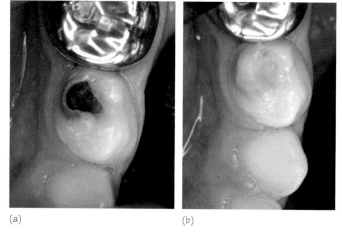

(a)　　　　　　　　　　　(b)

Figure 23.4 Occlusal lesions deemed as low risk of infection (a) can be restored using ART approach (b).

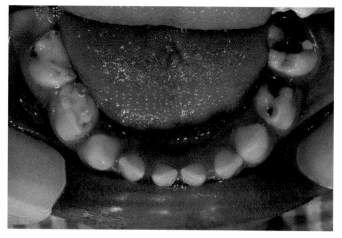

Figure 23.5 Patient with multiple carious lesions which have arrested. These can be restored using ART approach as shown on the right lower first and second primary molars.

Paediatric Dentistry at a Glance, First Edition. Monty Duggal, Angus Cameron and Jack Toumba. © 2013 John Wiley & Sons Ltd. Published 2013 by Blackwell Publishing Ltd.

Philosophy of care

Unfortunately many preschool children still have multiple extractions of decayed primary teeth under GA. Caries in the primary teeth is often ignored or treated poorly with glass ionomer cements without adequate treatment planning or regard to principles of restorative dentistry. Inevitably then many of these children develop pain or sepsis (Fig. 23.1) and are referred on to hospitals for the removal of carious and poorly restored primary molars under general anaesthesia. This treatment, though solving the immediate problem for the child, does not contribute positively to the child's dental health attitudes for the future and can lead to fear of dental procedures. Also, many children who have carious primary teeth thus extracted return a few years later with carious first permanent molars, many times necessitating a repeat general anaesthesia for their removal. Young children who present to dentists with extensive caries deserve highest quality care, which should have prevention at the heart, but also rehabilitation of the decayed dentition wherever possible, using the best restorative techniques. Treating caries effectively in pre-schoolers would improve the quality of life of millions of children.

Treatment planning

Relief from pain

Many children first attend the dentist with pain. Providing relief from toothache should be a priority. This may involve extraction of the unrestorable teeth. Stabilising the dentition with gentle excavation of open cavities and dressing with glass ionomers is often helpful.

Diagnosis

The root cause of the child having multiple carious lesions is established.

Preventive care

This should form the anchor of any treatment plan in children with extensive caries.

Rational restorative care

• Decision whether this can be provided with LA with or without sedation, or GA.
• In young children with extensive and multiple carious lesions a decision is made as to which teeth should be restored and which should be extracted. A **heroic treatment plan** to restore all teeth in a very young child is often misdirected, doomed to failure and not in the best interest of the child. For example, when all primary teeth are carious, it might be prudent to restore the second primary molars and extract the first primary molars (Fig. 23.2). Every treatment plan should be tailor made for the individual child, depending upon the diagnosis, and the child's behavioural and social history.
• In a child with extensive caries, full coverage with stainless steel or aesthetic crowns should be preferred.

The use of atraumatic restorative technique (ART)

This is a useful way to stabilise the carious dentition while a full treatment plan is drawn up and final restorative care is provided.

Sometimes poor restorations in primary molars have been clothed in a respectable garb (ART) (Fig. 23.3), which is described as a conservative procedure where some caries is removed without local analgesia and then a restoration such as glass ionomer is placed on top. Although this technique has some limited application in the practice of paediatric dentistry, mainly in areas with poor access to conventional restorative care, it should not be considered as a routine method for restoration of primary molars. Although a reasonable survival has been reported for occlusal restorations, extremely poor results are consistently reported for proximal cavities with over two thirds of the restorations lost over a 12–24-month period. The use of ART approach to multi-surface restorations should not be considered routinely.

Indications for use of ART

• As an interim restoration of carious primary teeth in pre-cooperative children.
• Only for teeth with low risk of pain and infection, mainly on caries affecting occlusal surfaces (Fig. 23.4).
• Restoration of arrested caries (Fig. 23.5).
• Temporary stabilisation of the dentition until definitive treatment is carried out.

Restoration of a large proximal cavity – indirect pulp capping (IPC)

One of the reasons for frequent failures associated with placing proximal restorations in extensively decayed primary molars is that pulp inflammation sets in early for proximal caries, and precedes the exposure of the pulp. Indirect pulp capping should only be carried out in such situations if the patient has been free of any symptoms of pulpitis or if a certain diagnosis of reversible pulpitis can be made. In all other situations a pulpotomy should be considered even if the pulp is not considered to be clinically exposed.

Indications for indirect pulp capping

• Deep cavity but a certain diagnosis of reversible pulpitis.
• Low caries risk children with low caries activity and caries attack rate.
• No history of previous abscesses.

In children where the caries activity and attack rate is high, a more radical approach should be taken. For example for a deep proximal cavity in a child with rampant caries, poor compliance, and with a history of previous abscesses, a pulpotomy rather than an indirect pulp capping should be carried out for a deep proximal cavity to avoid failure. Pulp responses for occlusal caries are milder as compared with proximal caries (Chapter 20), so indirect pulp capping is more successful for deep occlusal caries as compared to proximal. When IPC is carried out, protection of the pulp with a good material (e.g. GIC) and a good coronal seal preferably with SSC is essential.

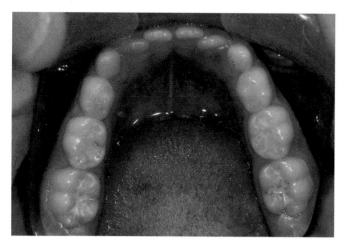

Figure 24.1 Opaque fissure sealant of mandibular first permanent molar teeth.

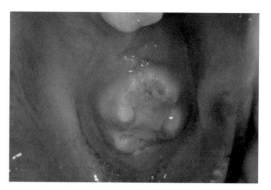

Figure 24.2 Maxillary left first permanent molar fissure sealed with a glass ionomer cement (GIC).

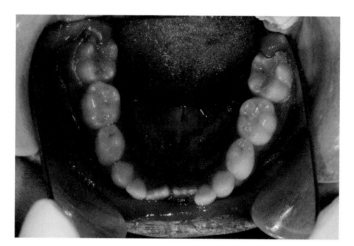

Figure 24.3 Partially erupted mandibular first permanent molars fissure sealed with GIC.

Paediatric Dentistry at a Glance, First Edition. Monty Duggal, Angus Cameron and Jack Toumba. © 2013 John Wiley & Sons Ltd. Published 2013 by Blackwell Publishing Ltd.

Protecting the first permanent molar

The first permanent molar teeth can be protected before, during and after their eruption into the oral cavity. It is therefore important to have established a safe oral environment into which these teeth will erupt and be maintained in for the future. Instilling intensive preventive measures is paramount to ensure that these teeth remain caries-free. The first permanent molar is most susceptible to developing dental caries within the first 2 years after eruption.

Prior to eruption
- Regular and effective good oral hygiene practices.
- Establishing good dietary regimes.
- Regular daily fluoride applications from tooth brushing and additional products as indicated depending on caries risk assessment.

During eruption
- Maintaining oral hygiene and dietary practices.
- Fissure sealing at-risk teeth (especially first permanent molars) as soon as possible on eruption depending on caries risk.
- Use of glass ionomer cements (GIC) for sealing first permanent molars which are partially erupted in individuals at risk of caries.

Post-eruption
- Maintaining oral hygiene and dietary practices.
- Careful monitoring and review of all teeth is essential to ensure that there is no new caries development or progression of lesions.

Use of fluorides
Chapters 11–14 on preventive care and fluorides give more information on the use of fluorides for caries prevention:
- twice daily brushing with toothpastes containing 1000–1450 ppm F;
- daily fluoride rinse (225 ppm F);
- fluoride varnish (22 600 ppm F) professional applications 2–4 times yearly.

Fissure sealants
Fissure sealants have been used to prevent occlusal caries in first permanent molars for over 50 years. Bisphenol-α-glycidyl methacrylate (bis-GMA) resin is the most effective sealant. The caries preventive success of sealants is due to the establishment of a tight seal, which prevents microleakage of nutrients to the microflora in the deeper parts of the pits and fissures.

Types
- Unfilled and filled.
- Clear, coloured and opaque.
- Chemical and light cured.

Indications
They are indicated for children that are assessed as being at risk of developing dental caries. The teeth should be sealed as soon as possible after eruption (Fig. 24.1) and carefully monitored and re-sealed or repaired as necessary. The following are indications for placing sealants:
- history of caries in primary dentition;
- caries in one or more first permanent molar;
- siblings with history of caries;
- special needs children – medical, physical, social or intellectual disabilities;
- mild hypoplastic molars;
- teeth with deep pits and fissures;
- as part of a preventive resin restoration.

Effectiveness
Resin-based sealants are the material of choice and have been shown to have the best success. Success rates for caries prevention have been reported to range from about 90% at 1 year to 50% at 5 years. It is very important to follow up sealed teeth both clinically and radiographically as they are prone to failure. Any partial loss should be repaired and lost sealants replaced. There is a 5–10% failure rate per year so that the retention rates decline with time from 75–80% at 2 years to 50% at 4 years. Salivary contamination due to poor moisture control at placement is the main cause of sealant failure. GIC can be used as a sealant in partially erupted first permanent molars (Figs. 24.2 and 24.3). One particular GIC sealant is Fuji Triage, which is a pink GIC sealant. It has many advantages. Firstly it can be applied where isolation is poor due to the first permanent molar being partially erupted or in a child with poor cooperation. Secondly, due to its pink colour it can be easily visualised and when it is no longer visible on the occlusal surface a conventional sealant can then be placed.

Technique
1. **Isolation:** with rubber dam or cotton wool rolls.
2. **Surface preparation:** cleaning or polishing beforehand has not been shown to be more beneficial than the effect of acid etching alone. Some advocate the use of rotating burs to remove superficial enamel to allow better penetration of the resin into the fissure. Orthophosphoric acid (37%) etchant is used as an etchant for at least 15 seconds.
3. **Rinsing and drying:** irrigation with water spray for 30 seconds and drying with uncontaminated compressed air for 15 seconds.
4. **Sealant placement:** the key to success is not to use an excessive amount of sealant beyond the etched area otherwise microleakage will occur and sealant retention will be compromised.
5. **Review:** careful clinical and radiographic monitoring is needed. Any loss of sealant must be repaired or replaced.

Guidelines
A number of guidelines from professional bodies and academies are available for fissure sealants. These can help and guide dental practitioners on the use of fissure sealants in children.

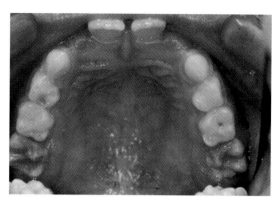

Figure 25.1 Intra-oral photograph of upper arch showing hypomineralised upper first permanent molars.

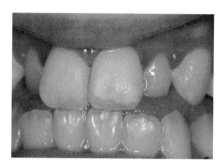

Figure 25.2 Intra-oral photograph showing demarcated opacities on an incisor, typical of MIH.

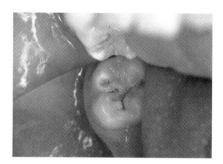

Figure 25.3 Enamel which is hypomineralised tends to break off after eruption, also known as posteruptive loss of enamel.

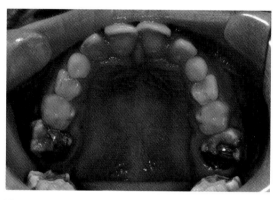

Figure 25.4 Atypical restorations of first permanent molars. Many dentists do not recognise this condition and try to treat it as they would a carious lesion.

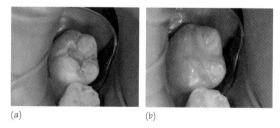

(a)   (b)

Figure 25.5 Showing a demarcated area of hypomineralisation on occlusal surface (a) being prepared for composite restoration (b).

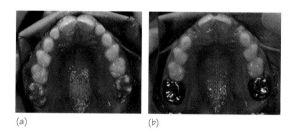

(a)   (b)

Figure 25.6 Hypomineralised upper first permanent molars (a) restored with SSCs (b).

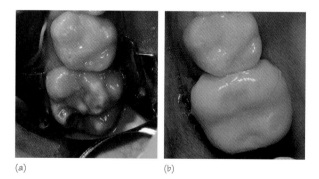

(a)   (b)

Figure 25.7 Hypomineralised upper first permanent molar (a) restored with ProTemp® crown (b).

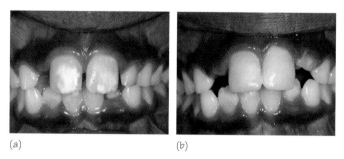

(a)   (b)

Figure 25.8 Demarcated opacity on upper incisors (a) treated with composite after removing half the thickness of the opacity and layering with an opaque shade followed by dentine and enamel shades to mask the defect (b).

Paediatric Dentistry at a Glance, First Edition. Monty Duggal, Angus Cameron and Jack Toumba. © 2013 John Wiley & Sons Ltd. Published 2013 by Blackwell Publishing Ltd.

Molar incisor hypomineralisation (MIH)/molar hypomineralisation (MH)

MIH is characterised by hypomineralised lesions on first permanent molars (FPMs) and incisors. If only FPMs are involved then the term MH is used. The hypomineralised lesions usually manifest as yellowish demarcated opacities on the affected teeth (Fig. 25.1). Prevalence in Europe is reported to be 6–14%.

Recognition

Children usually present with:
- demarcated opacities on molars and/or incisors (Fig. 25.2);
- posteruptive enamel loss (Fig. 25.3);
- atypical restorations on FPMs (Fig. 25.4);
- extraction of first permanent molars.

Differential diagnosis

It is important to differentiate MIH from other conditions manifest as hypomineralised disorders of enamel such as amelogenesis imperfecta (AI).

Aetiology

The aetiology is not completely understood so sometimes the term "idiopathic opacities" is still used. Most children with MIH presented with potential medical aetiological factors during the prenatal, perinatal and postnatal period. The majority of these conditions produce either hypocalcaemia, or hypoxia to child or mother. An association exists between the following conditions and MIH if these occur in the first few months of life:
- antibiotic use in first few months;
- ear infections;
- fevers in first year of life;
- perinatal conditions.

Clinical problems and their management

In addition to their other problems, children with MIH have behaviour management issues and increased dental fear and anxiety.

Sensitivity

This is the presenting feature in many cases. The affected teeth can be extremely sensitive so DO NOT blow cold air on them during examination. Sensitivity can be due to:
- porous enamel and exposed dentine due to posteruptive loss of enamel;
- underlying pulp inflammation can lead to peripheral sensitisation;
- extreme apprehension and anxiety compounds sensitivity.

Alleviation of sensitivity is difficult. It can be achieved with:
- restoration of lost tissue;
- regular applications of fluoride varnish;
- once daily use of casein phosphopeptide with amorphous calcium phosphate (tooth mousse), except in those with allergy to milk products.

Achieving profound analgesia

This is sometimes difficult to achieve. Some useful tips are:
- use articaine instead of lignocaine for infiltration;
- supplement the infiltration with intraligamental;
- inhalation sedation alleviates anxiety and provides some relative analgesia;
- use rubber dam isolation to protect other sensitive molars;
- DO NOT use high-volume suction.

Loss of tooth substance

Composite resins (Fig. 25.5) are used for:
- well demarcated defects confined to one or two surfaces;
- no cusp involvement;
- margins preferably supragingival;
- no significant sensitivity.

Stainless steel crowns (Fig. 25.6) are used for:
- extensive defects;
- maintenance of severely affected tooth essential;
- presence of sensitivity.

Sometimes aesthetic crowns for medium-term restoration can be performed using Protemp Crowns (3M ESPE) (Fig. 25.7). However, their longevity has not been studied in these situations.

Aesthetics

Many children are concerned about the appearance of the incisors due to the presence of opacity on the labial surface. These lesions are not always easy to mask. The following steps will give good results:

1. Using high speed and diamond bur remove about half the thickness of the opacity.

2. Use an opaque shade as first layer to achieve "masking" of the lesion.

3. Build up the remaining using appropriate dentine and enamel shades (Fig. 25.8).

For some superficial lesions microabrasion can also be useful.

Long-term management

A long-term treatment plan is required in order not to leave the child with heavily restored FPMs which will require lifelong restorative care or worse still extraction later in life. When FPMs are considered to have a poor prognosis:
- orthodontic opinion is sought;
- extraction of all first permanent molars is considered with due consideration to the timing that would facilitate eruption of the second permanent molars to replace the FPMs.

The best time for the extraction of the FPMs is when:
- the development of bifurcation of the second permanent molars is evident, usually at age of 8.5–9.5 years.
- there is some evidence of development of the third molar crypt.

For those teeth that have been restored with stainless steel crowns, long-term management with aesthetic crowns is offered at the appropriate age.

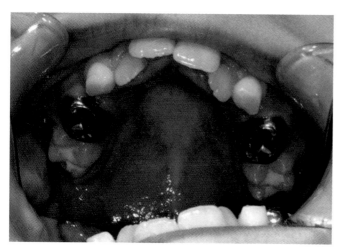

Figure 26.1 Space loss due to premature extraction of both upper first primary molars.

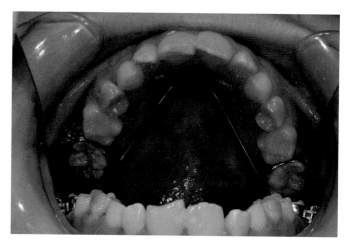

Figure 26.2 Nance appliance.

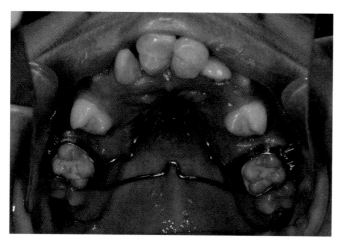

Figure 26.3 Transpalatal arch.

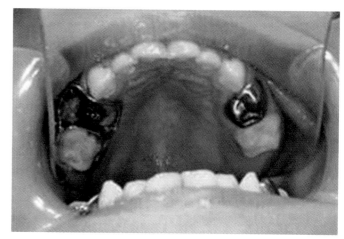

Figure 26.4 Band and loop space maintainer.

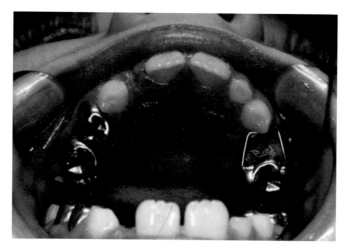

Figure 26.5 Crown and loop space maintainer.

Paediatric Dentistry at a Glance, First Edition. Monty Duggal, Angus Cameron and Jack Toumba. © 2013 John Wiley & Sons Ltd. Published 2013 by Blackwell Publishing Ltd.

Space management

Common orthodontic problems stem from crowding and the lack of space available for the permanent dentition to erupt. Usually the problem arises due to premature loss of the deciduous teeth from trauma, caries or pulp pathology (Fig. 26.1). Maintaining space is important and every effort should be made to preserve the primary teeth to prevent problems in the developing dentition such as space loss. However, space maintainers are not required every time a primary molar is lost prematurely. The decision to fit a space maintainer after enforced extraction must be arrived at by balancing the occlusal disturbance that may result against the plaque accumulation and caries that the appliance may cause and poor oral hygiene, which is a contraindication. A decision to fit a space maintainer should be made only after a careful assessment of the developing occlusion and its predicted patterns and the patient factors such as behaviour, compliance and oral hygiene.

Common causes of space loss in primary and mixed dentition

- Premature loss of primary teeth.
- Congenitally missing teeth.
- Unrestored proximal carious lesions.
- Ectopic eruption or permanent teeth.
- Ankylosis.
- Dental anomalies particularly microdontia (e.g. peg-shaped laterals).

Indications for space maintainers

These are most useful in two situations:
- Loss of a primary first molar where crowding is severe, i.e. more than 3.5 mm (half a unit) per quadrant. In this situation space loss due to drift may be so severe that the extraction of one premolar may be insufficient to relieve resultant crowding so that subsequent orthodontic treatment is more difficult.
- Loss of a primary second molar, except in spaced arches.

Other indications are:
- loss of permanent upper incisors;
- delayed eruption of permanent central incisors due to presence of supernumerary;
- maintaining first premolar space (after extraction of first primary molar) for unerupted permanent canines;
- where crowding would be expected.

Space maintainers should be used only where adequate space is available for its placement (well aligned/uncrowded arches) and also where space closure would otherwise take place.

Contraindications for space maintainers

- Uncooperative patients, poor compliance.
- Poor oral hygiene.
- High caries risk/susceptibility.
- Where malocclusion is unavoidable.
- Sufficient size of dental base for size of teeth.
- Hypodontia.
- Where premolars are about to erupt.

Treatment planning considerations

- Patient's cooperation and tolerance to the space maintainer (the shorter period, the better). This should also include the parents' cooperation and motivation, as well as the patient's overall dental compliance.

- Length (antero-posterior) of dental base and tooth : tissue ratio. If there is sufficient space for the second and third molars mesial drift of the molars would not be expected. For patients with very short dental bases, crowding is usually unavoidable and, hence, the use of space maintainers is limited in such cases. Patients with long dental bases would have problems in persisting extraction spaces, not loss of space.
- Dental age. This is a more important consideration than the chronological age. Need to assess eruption sequence and root formation in order to predict eruption of permanent teeth.
- Pre-existing occlusion.
- Eruption sequence.
- Presence and root development of permanent successor.
- Amount of alveolar bone covering permanent successor. An estimation of 6 months should be anticipated for every millimetre of bone coverage.
- Patient's medical history, oral habits, hygiene.

Therefore, a proper pre-treatment assessment should be done while planning for a space maintainer. In addition to a complete clinical examination, a full radiographic assessment, study models and a mixed dentition analysis are necessary.

Types of space maintainers

A number of designs of removable appliances are possible but these are not preferred due to poor patient compliance. Fixed space maintainers designs are:
- distal shoe – historic, seldom made as difficult to construct and poorly tolerated;
- Nance appliance – upper arch only (Fig. 26.2);
- transpalatal arch – upper arch only (Fig. 26.3);
- crown and loop – both upper and lower arch (Fig. 26.4);
- band and loop (Fig. 26.5);
- lingual arch – only in lower arch.

Advantages

- Prevent drifting of neighbouring teeth, especially if permanent successor is not expected to erupt within the next 6 months.
- Enables the "leeway space" to be used in cases where there is just enough space.

Disadvantages

- Cannot predict the need for active orthodontic treatment in the future, so space prediction is educated guess work!
- Risk of irritation to oral tissues especially if worn for long periods.
- Higher risk of plaque accumulation and caries.

Follow-up care

If the space maintainer is required for more than 6 months, and particularly if the first permanent molar is banded, it is advisable to remove the space maintainer every 3–4 months and apply fluoride to the surface of the teeth. The frequency of fluoride application can be increased or decreased depending on the assessment of the patient's caries risk.

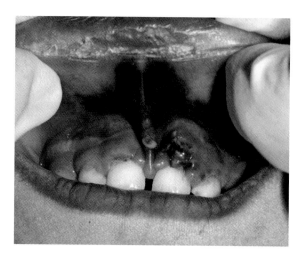

Figure 27.1 Soft tissue injury to the labial fraenum. This is a common injury and non-accidental injury should not be discounted.

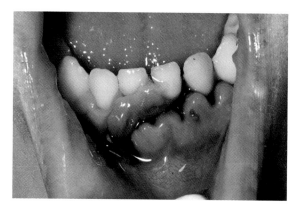

Figure 27.2 Gingival laceration and degloving from blunt trauma.

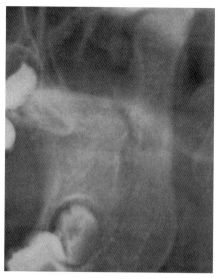

Figure 27.3 Subcondylar fracture of the mandible – the most common facial fracture found in children.

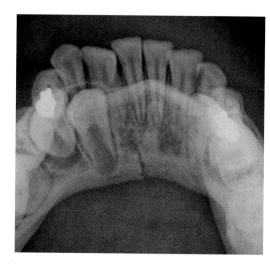

Figure 27.4 A parasymphyseal fracture with minimal displacement. Many of the fractures in children are "greenstick" and present with minimal or no displacement.

Table 27.1 Paediatric Glasgow Coma Score (children >1 year).

Eye opening	
Spontaneously	4
To speech	3
To pain	2
None	1
Verbal	
Conversant and uses appropriate words	5
Confused and uses inappropriate words	4
Cries persistently to pain	3
Incomprehensible sounds or moans to pain	2
None	1
Motor	
Obeys commands	6
Localises pain	5
Withdraws from pain	4
Abnormal flexion to pain	3
Abnormal extension to pain	2
None	1

Severity of head injury: <9 severe, 9–12 moderate, 13–15 mild.
Modified from Teasdale G, Jennett B (1974) Assessment of coma and impaired consciousness: a practical scale. Lancet 304: 81–84.

Paediatric Dentistry at a Glance, First Edition. Monty Duggal, Angus Cameron and Jack Toumba. © 2013 John Wiley & Sons Ltd. Published 2013 by Blackwell Publishing Ltd.

Frequency of trauma in children

- 30% suffer injury to the primary dentition.
- 22% injure their permanent teeth.
- Peak incidence 2–4 years and then at 8–10 years.
- Male : female ratio, 2 : 1.
- Overjet 3–6 mm – twice the frequency of trauma; >6 mm – threefold increase.

Child management

It is important to assess early how the child is going to cope with the required treatment. In the emergency situation, it is easy to concentrate on all the procedures that are required and forget about appropriate child management and the concerns of the parents.

- Can the child cope with the procedure?
- Non-pharmacological behaviour management techniques.
- Pharmacological techniques:
  - relative analgesia;
  - sedation – oral, nasal, rectal, IV;
  - general anaesthesia.

Principles of primary care

It is essential to take the time to take a thorough history and completely examine the child. This is especially important in assessing long-term prognosis and may be important in litigation.

- Accurate history:
  - Are there any medical co-morbidities?
  - Did the child sustain any other injuries?
  - Was there a loss of consciousness?
  - Prognosis of injuries.
  - Litigation.
- Thorough examination of the head and neck and any other areas that sustained trauma. Examine both extra-oral and intra-oral.

History

Questions to ask:
- When and how did the trauma occur?
- Were there any other injuries sustained?
- What initial treatment was given?
- Have there been other dental injuries in the past?
- Is the child fully immunised against tetanus?

Examination

- Extra-oral:
  - facial skeleton, skull and facial bones;
  - soft tissues - lacerations, grazing etc. (Figs. 27.1 and 27.2);
  - assessment of cranial nerves.
- Intra-oral:
  - soft tissues - lacerations, degloving;
  - fractures or displacement of bone;
  - displacement and damage to teeth;
  - alterations in the occlusion;
  - mobility, pulp exposure, percussion;
  - pulp sensibility testing.

Investigations

Radiographs

As it is often difficult to obtain diagnostic intra-oral radiographs from an injured young child there is advantage in using extra-oral panoramic radiographs. When determining the presence of a root fracture, several films may be required at different angulations.

Dento-alveolar injuries:
- periapical films;
- panoramic radiographs.

Mandibular fracture/condylar head fracture:
- panoramic radiographs;
- cone-beam tomography/computed tomography (CT) scan;
- true mandibular occlusal.

Maxillary fractures:
- CT scan.

Pulp sensibility tests

Always record a baseline assessment of pulpal status, but the initial response may be unreliable. Of all the available tests, thermal sensitivity is the most reproducible and most accurate.

Percussion tests

Percussion tests are of great value in determining apical inflammation. While colour change and the other tests mentioned above are important, a previously traumatised tooth that is tender to percussion usually indicates pulp necrosis.

Facial fractures (Figs. 27.3 and 27.4)

In children 70% of all facial fractures involve the condyle. While rare, other fractures do not typically follow the classical Le Fort lines that might be seen in adults. Treatment is conservative with regard to the developing dentition and growth considerations. Signs to consider include:
- facial asymmetry and ecchymosis or a sublingual haematoma;
- subconjunctival haematoma and/or tethering of the globe;
- strabismus and diplopia;
- CSF rhinorrhoea and epistaxis;
- occlusal discrepancies, intra-oral mucosal tears and lacerations;
- anaesthesia or paraesthesia of infraorbital or mental nerve;
- pain, swelling, stepping and limitation of jaw movement.

Head injury in children (Table 27.1)

The identification of head injury in children is critically important and any child who loses consciousness needs medical assessment:
- loss or altered states of consciousness;
- persistent headache that worsens over time;
- vomiting;
- swelling on the scalp or bleeding from the scalp;
- seizure or convulsions, disorientation or confusion;
- dysarthria, dysphasia or dysphagia, altered vision or diplopia;
- a fall from greater than 2 m;
- CSF leakage or bleeding from nose or ears.

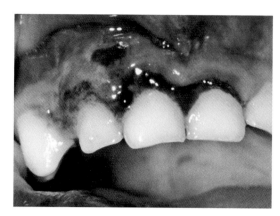

Figure 28.1 Luxation of the upper anterior teeth with minimal displacement. There has been some gingival disruption but essentially no treatment is required.

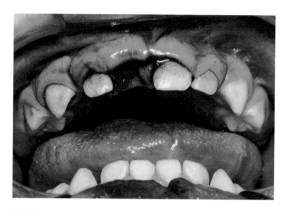

Figure 28.2 Intrusive luxation of the upper right primary incisor. On a cursory examination, it might appear that the tooth has been lost but there has been expansion of the labial plate. Intrusions are some of the most common injuries in young children. A periapical or true lateral maxillary radiograph is required to assess the relationship of the primary incisor to the permanent tooth. In many cases these teeth will re-erupt.

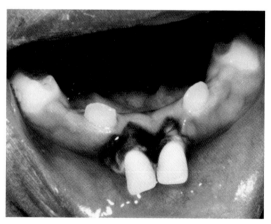

Figure 28.3 In the lower arch, a luxation of the primary incisors is usually towards the labial. These teeth should not be repositioned as it is likely that the roots will be forced posteriorly into the developing permanent incisors.

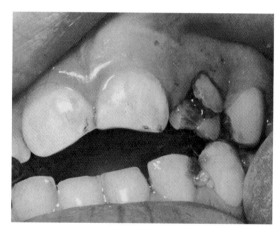

Figure 28.4 A vertical root fracture of an upper left primary lateral incisor. Unfortunately, these teeth are unrestorable and need extraction.

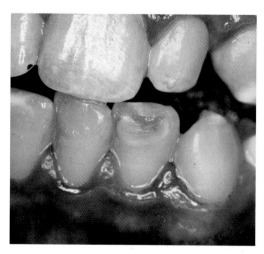

Figure 28.5 An isolated enamel defect caused by intrusion of lower primary incisor into the crown of the lower permanent lateral incisor.

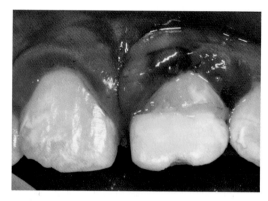

Figure 28.6 A more severe complication following trauma to the primary incisors. This is a dilaceration of the crown and the root of the permanent tooth with a hypoplastic defect involving the gingival margin. These are difficult to restore adequately and usually require a gingival procedure to expose the damaged cervical area of the crown.

Paediatric Dentistry at a Glance, First Edition. Monty Duggal, Angus Cameron and Jack Toumba. © 2013 John Wiley & Sons Ltd. Published 2013 by Blackwell Publishing Ltd.

Frequency and aetiology

Trauma in young children is extremely common with up to 30% of children suffering injuries to their primary teeth. It is obviously upsetting for parents. The peak incidence is at 2–4 years of age when children are toddlers and still learning gross motor skills. Falls and play accidents are the most common cause of injuries. While child abuse contributes only a small percentage of injuries, those treating children should be aware of children presenting with injuries that are inconsistent with the history and be prepared to inform their appropriate child protection authorities about such incidents. It is important to remember that the responsibility of the clinician is to the child first and not the alleged perpetrator. Dog bites account for a significant number of injuries, and, commonly, the animal is known to the child.

Assessment

There must be a thorough history and examination of the child to exclude any other injures or medical conditions that might affect your management. The treating dentist also needs to be cognisant of the concerns of the child and those of the parents about the immediate treatment needs and possible long-term sequelae for the permanent dentition. At this time it is essential to consider what behaviour management techniques might be required and it is appropriate that sedation or general anaesthesia might be needed for many young children requiring invasive treatment.

Luxations in the primary dentition

In most cases, there are only two options in management; either to extract the traumatised tooth or leave it alone and observe. Repositioning of displaced primary teeth runs the risk of further damage to the permanent successor. While it is possible to splint luxated primary teeth, there are always difficulties in placing the splint in a traumatised young child, and then having to remove it later! Warn parents about the risk of tooth discolouration and possible pulp necrosis. Always check the immunisation status, begin a soft diet and give advice to parents regarding possible sequelae.

Concussion and subluxation

In these cases there is no displacement of the primary tooth but increased mobility and possible gingival damage (Fig. 28.1). The tooth will be tender to bite on and a soft diet and follow-up are all that is required. A periapical radiograph will confirm the presence of any root fracture.

Intrusive and lateral luxations (Fig. 28.2)

Perhaps the most common of all the injuries, intrusion of a primary incisor has the potential to cause the most damage to the permanent successor. A true lateral maxillary radiograph is useful to determine the extent of the vertical displacement and the relation of the primary tooth apex to the permanent incisor. If the crown is still visible and there is minimal alveolar damage, then the tooth will usually re-erupt. If totally intruded, then the tooth should be extracted. Soft tissues should be sutured if required.

Extrusive luxations (Fig. 28.3)

Teeth that are minimally displaced and not excessively mobile may be retained, but otherwise, these teeth should be extracted. It is uncommon in these cases to have significant soft tissue damage.

Avulsion

Avulsed primary teeth should NOT be replanted. Replanting these teeth may significantly damage the permanent tooth due to displacement of the blood clot into the developing follicle. Unless there is significant soft tissue damage (requiring suturing), no other treatment is required.

Fractures
Uncomplicated fractures

In the young pre-cooperative child, very little treatment is required other than smoothing sharp edges. Remember that, by the time a primary tooth exfoliates at age 6–7 years, up to half of the clinical crown of a primary tooth may be lost by normal attrition. In older, more compliant patients, these teeth may be restored.

Complicated crown/root fractures (Fig. 28.4)

All too commonly, a complicated fracture extends below the gingival margin and these teeth often have several fractures through the root. These teeth are essentially unrestorable and should be removed. In many cases, the tooth is shattered into multiple fragments, making a normally simple extraction very difficult in a young child. Avoid any further damage to the permanent teeth by excessive elevation of tooth fragments.

Root fractures

In those teeth where the root fracture is in the apical half and there is minimal mobility, then the tooth may be retained. If the coronal fragment has been displaced and is mobile then this should be removed. The apical portion invariably retains its vitality and there should be no attempt at extracting this for risk of damaging the permanent tooth.

Dento-alveolar fractures

In the lower arch, primary incisors are commonly displaced anteriorly as a dento-alveolar fragment comprising labial plate and teeth. If the teeth are to be removed, then it is important to preserve the labial plate of bone, otherwise the whole segment can be repositioned and sutured in place. There are rarely complications with the permanent teeth that are sitting lingual to the lower incisors.

Sequelae following primary trauma

- Pulp necrosis with grey discolouration and/or abscess formation.
- Internal resorption (pink discoloration).
- Ankylosis of primary tooth.
- Hypoplasia or hypomineralisation of permanent successor.
- Dilaceration of crown and/or root (Figs. 28.5 and 28.6).
- Resorption of permanent tooth germ (rare).

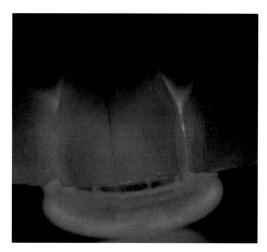

Figure 29.1 Transillumination to observe cracks and infractions in the enamel following trauma.

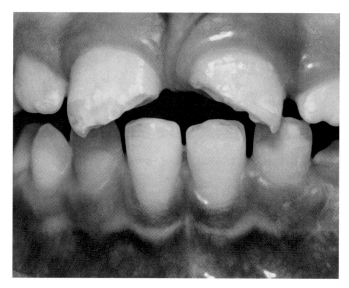

Figure 29.2 Proximal fractures in a young child without pulp exposure.

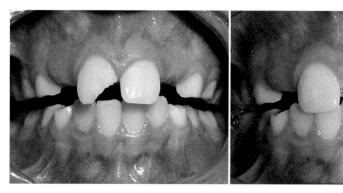

Figure 29.3 Composite resin is a perfect material in children and adolescents for the restoration of anterior teeth. It provides good strength and aesthetics and can be quickly and simply placed. Advanced restorative options should not be considered until the child has finished growth. When restoring these traumatised teeth it is essential that the restoration has adequate bulk of material to support itself in function.

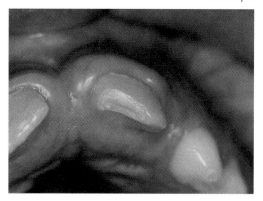

Figure 29.4 A typical presentation of a mesial proximal fracture of a young permanent incisor. It is important to cover the exposed dentine as soon as possible to prevent pulp necrosis. These immature teeth have wide-open dentinal tubules and should be protected in the interim with a glass ionomer cement prior to restoration of the crown with composite resin.

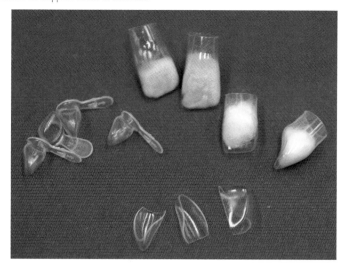

Figure 29.5 Strip crowns and incisal corners aid in restoring anterior teeth with composite resin.

Paediatric Dentistry at a Glance, First Edition. Monty Duggal, Angus Cameron and Jack Toumba. © 2013 John Wiley & Sons Ltd. Published 2013 by Blackwell Publishing Ltd.

Infractions

An infraction represents a crack in the enamel without the loss of any tooth structure. It is best diagnosed with the use of transillumination (Fig. 29.1), shining a high-intensity light from the palatal surface of tooth. There is a low risk of subsequent pulp necrosis independent of any other injuries such as luxation.

Management

- Pulp sensibility test at presentation.
- Periapical radiograph.
- Warn parents and child about the risk of pulp necrosis.
- Review at 3 months and then 12 months.

Pulp sensibility tests

Children will often give false responses to pulp sensibility testing especially early after a traumatic event. Furthermore, they may respond to the pressure of the test rather than the sensation of cold or electrical stimulation. Recently traumatised teeth will often fail to respond normally initially after the injury but this should not be taken to indicate pulp necrosis.

- Begin testing on a normal tooth.
- Cold tests are usually easier to interpret in younger children than electrical tests.
- Try testing the tooth with pressure first (turn the ice stick around so that there is no cold sensation only the touch).
- Use multiple tests and then test other teeth before returning to the traumatised tooth.

Uncomplicated fractures

An uncomplicated enamel (class I Ellis) or enamel/dentine (class II Ellis) fracture does not involve the pulp (Fig. 29.2). The aim of management is the preservation of pulp vitality. It is important to remember that recently erupted permanent incisors have wide-open dentinal tubules and there is an increased risk of pulp necrosis as the size of the fracture increases. Generally, there is a low risk of pulp necrosis (~3.5%), however, with large proximal fractures this may increase to 54% (Ravn, 1981). Protective coverage of the dentine may reduce this risk to 8%. Good practice, therefore, dictates that children suffering these injuries should be seen as early as possible and any exposed dentine covered with a glass ionomer cement. It is often preferable to delay placement of the final restoration.

Management

- Baseline periapical radiographs and pulp sensibility tests.
- Enamel-only fractures may only require smoothing with a disc or may be restored with composite resin.
- Enamel/dentine – cover dentine initially and then restore with composite resin (Fig. 29.3). It is not essential that the tooth is restored immediately, but it is important to protect the dentine and the pulp (Fig. 29.4).
- Review at 3, 6 and 12 months with pulp sensibility tests and radiographs at 12 months.

Tips for restoring fractured incisal corners

- Prepare enamel with a broad chamfer. This allows for maximum bonding of the composite resin to enamel prisms perpendicularly while achieving a butt-joint finishing margin.
- Avoid long bevels with a feather-edge finish, the margins of which will fail over time with chipping.
- Cover dentine with a thin layer of glass ionomer base.
- Prefabricated cellulose–acetate incisal corners are extremely useful (Fig. 29.5).
- Choose the shade and translucency of composite resin carefully as the enamel of newly erupted incisors is often more opaque than that seen in older patients.
- Incremental build-ups with dentine and enamel shades ensure excellent colour and translucency matching.
- Class IV composite resin build-ups must have an adequate bulk of material to give strength and longevity to the restoration.
- Preserve fractured enamel pieces as these can be recemented to the crown. It is often easier to reattach these pieces rather than trying to match colour and form using composite resin.

Always protect the dentine following trauma.

Complicated crown fractures

Complicated fractures of enamel and dentine involve the pulp tissue and every effort must be made to prevent pulp necrosis. This is especially the case when managing those teeth with immature, open apices, where the consequence of a non-vital pulp severely compromises the long-term prognosis of the tooth. A pulp exposed to the oral cavity cannot heal and the outcome of an untreated complicated crown fracture is pulp necrosis. Unfortunately, there is little evidence in the literature as to how long an exposed pulp can survive, so these children should be managed as quickly as possible.

Management

Management aim – to preserve vital, non-inflamed pulp tissue, biologically walled off by a hard tissue barrier.

- Early assessment and treatment.
- Periapical radiographs at different horizontal angulations to exclude root fractures (see Chapter 32).

Complete root apex with vital pulp

- If the period of exposure is short and vital tissue is still present, then a partial pulpotomy (Cvek) may be performed at any level on teeth with closed apices. The procedure for Cvek pulpotomy is discussed in Chapter 30.
- Preserving part of the pulp is always preferable to performing root canal therapy.
- If there are restorative considerations, such as the need for a post or support for a crown, then root canal therapy may be required.

Complete root apex with necrotic pulp

- Commence root canal therapy.

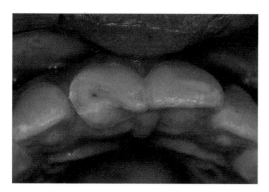

Figure 30.1 Proximal fracture on the upper right central incisor with an immature apex.

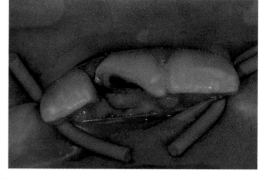

Figure 30.2 Cvek pulpotomy procedure. Isolation with rubber dam and local anaesthesia; 1–2 mm of pulpal tissue has been removed down to vital bleeding pulp.

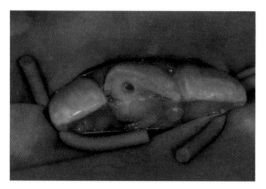

Figure 30.3 Cessation of pulpal bleeding with copious irrigation with saline. It is essential that there is no blood clot left over the amputated pulp surface. The medicament will be placed directly over this cut surface.

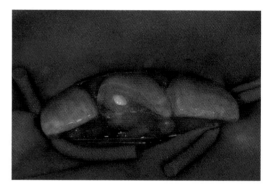

Figure 30.4 A non-setting calcium hydroxide base is placed followed by a setting base prior to restoration of the tooth.

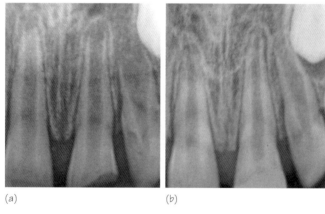

(a)   (b)

Figure 30.5 Apexogenesis following a Cvek pulpotomy. The upper left central incisor (a) has an immature apex.

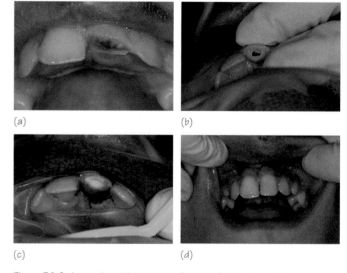

(a)   (b)

(c)   (d)

Figure 30.6 A complicated crown root fracture (a) treated with a coronal pulpotomy with the removal of entire coronal pulp (b). The fracture line was exposed with electrosurgery (c) and tooth restored with composite resin (d).

Paediatric Dentistry at a Glance, First Edition. Monty Duggal, Angus Cameron and Jack Toumba. © 2013 John Wiley & Sons Ltd. Published 2013 by Blackwell Publishing Ltd.

Rationale for management of incisors with incomplete root development and vital pulp

Continued root development in immature traumatised incisors depends upon pulp healing. If the pulp becomes non-vital, root development will cease. Incomplete root development will mean that there is insufficient amount of dentine and cementum, and also an inadequate crown : root ratio, leaving the root structure inherently weak and at risk of root fracture under masticatory forces. A wide root canal with an open apex also creates an endodontic challenge for the clinician. Therefore, all attempts must be made to carry out treatments to facilitate pulp healing which will allow normal and continued root development, thereby vastly improving the prognosis of the traumatised teeth (Fig. 30.1).

Management options to facilitate pulp healing

Pulp capping

This should be considered in very few cases specifically for very small uncontaminated exposures that have presented almost immediately after the trauma to the dentist.

The following should be performed:

1. Administer local analgesia and use rubber dam.
2. Irrigate dentine and exposed pulp gently with saline to wash off any superficial contamination.
3. Apply a thin layer of non-setting calcium hydroxide to the exposure site, completely covering the exposed pulp.
4. Apply a thin layer of glass ionomer cement over the calcium hydroxide.
5. Restore the crown with composite resin to ensure a complete coronal seal.

Follow-up care

Regular follow up should be performed to monitor:
• reaction of pulp to sensibility tests, both thermal and electric;
• colour change;
• continued root development;
• patient symptoms that might indicate the pulp is not healing.

Pulpotomy

Pulp capping is not preferred after trauma unless the exposure is very small, uncontaminated and the patient presents immediately after trauma.

The aim of carrying out a pulpotomy is the removal of the pulp that might be contaminated, leaving behind uncontaminated healthy pulp that can then heal, and root development can continue as normal. Depending upon the length of exposure and the extent of contamination the following techniques have been suggested:
• partial (Cvek's) pulpotomy;
• coronal pulpotomy;
• corono-radicular pulpotomy.

The Cvek or "partial pulpotomy" procedure involves the removal of contaminated pulpal tissue and placement of a calcium hydroxide dressing over the amputated, uncontaminated, vital tissue to allow preservation of vitality in the remaining pulp and thereby continued development of the tooth root and closure of the apex. This procedure has excellent success and should be performed as soon after the trauma as possible.

Partial/Cvek pulpotomy procedure (Figs. 30.2, 30.3 and 30.4)

1. Local anaesthesia and rubber dam are always required.
2. Remove 1–2 mm or more of pulp tissue with a clean diamond bur until vital bleeding tissue is reached.
3. Irrigate the exposed pulp with sterile saline until bleeding stops but do not leave any blood clot present. Local anaesthetic solution may also be used, but do not inject directly into the pulp.
4. Place a non-setting calcium hydroxide dressing over the vital tissue. It is essential that this dressing is placed directly over the pulp and that no blood clot remains.
5. Cover with a setting calcium hydroxide base and then a glass ionomer to seal the access cavity.
6. Restore the tooth with composite resin.
7. Review at 6–8 weeks and then at 12 months with radiographs to monitor development of a hard tissue barrier and continued root development (Fig. 30.5).

Coronal or corono-radicular pulpotomy procedure

This is similar to the one described above with the difference being in the level of pulp amputation. If the extent of contamination is deemed to be severe, the entire pulp in the pulp chamber (coronal pulpotomy) or even deeper into the root canal (corono-radicular pulpotomy) can be removed until normal bleeding is evident. It is important to restore the fractured crown and ensure that the remaining pulp is protected from further insult and allowed to heal (Fig. 30.6).

Healing after pulpotomy

The following types of healing can be seen:
• continued root development and normal closure of apex;
• pulp canal obliteration. Seen often and sometimes complete sclerosis and obliteration of root canal can be seen. However, this is a sign of pulp healing as most teeth will remain vital. Pulp canal obliteration is not an indication for initiating root canal treatment for the tooth.

Follow-up care after pulpotomy

Pulpotomised teeth should be reviewed both clinically and with radiographs on a regular basis. Clinically, observe for colour change, tenderness to palpation and percussion and any symptoms reported by the patient. Radiographic evaluation should be carried out 4-monthly in the first year and followed by every 6 months in the second year. If there is no evidence of continued root development or any signs or symptoms that suggest irreversible pulp inflammation or necrosis, endodontic treatment is commenced immediately.

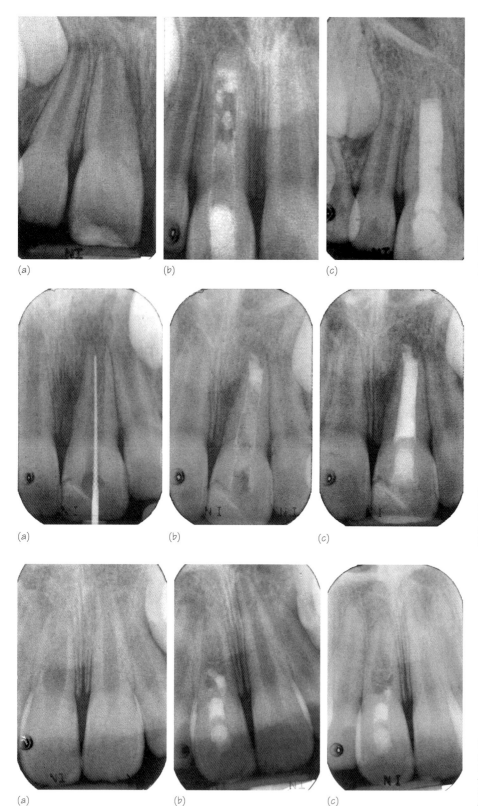

Figure 31.1 Apexification. This immature tooth became necrotic (a) and required apexification (b) to form an apex against which the gutta percha obturation could be condensed (c). Unfortunately, these teeth are very brittle across the cervical area and are prone to root fracture.

(a)   (b)   (c)

Figure 31.2 Periapical radiographs of upper left central incisor before (a) and after application of MTA to form an apical barrier (b) and after obturation with thermoplasticised gutta percha (c).

(a)   (b)   (c)

Figure 31.3 Periapical radiograph showing non-vital upper left central incisor with incomplete root development (a) which was treated with regenerative endodontic technique (b). Note deposition of hard tissue around apices of the treated tooth 1 year after treatment (c).

(a)   (b)   (c)

Paediatric Dentistry at a Glance, First Edition. Monty Duggal, Angus Cameron and Jack Toumba. © 2013 John Wiley & Sons Ltd. Published 2013 by Blackwell Publishing Ltd.

Incomplete root development with necrotic pulp

When immature permanent incisors lose their vitality, incomplete root development poses the following challenges for the clinician:
• the root has thin dentine walls liable to fracture under physiological forces;
• a wide, open apex;
• wide root canal space which is time consuming and technically difficult to treat.

Endodontic procedures should aim to not only form a barrier at the apex against which the canal may be obturated but also strengthen the remaining root structure. Some 75% suffer root fracture within 5 years. Several options for treatment are available.

Apexification with calcium hydroxide

The **aim** of apexification is to create an apical hard tissue barrier against which a root canal filling can be placed, by using calcium hydroxide treatment (Fig. 31.1).

1. Local anaesthesia may or may not be required.
2. Place rubber dam and prepare traditional access cavity.
3. Extirpate necrotic tissue and chemo-mechanically prepare the canal 1 mm short of the radiographic apex, attempting to preserve as much root thickness as possible.
4. Spiral calcium hydroxide paste into the canal ensuring that the paste is well condensed and in contact with apical tissue.
5. Access cavity is restored with glass ionomer cement and the tooth restored with composite resin.
6. Review 3–6-monthly with radiographs and change/redress with calcium hydroxide if there is loss of the dressing in the canal.
7. The formation of a calcific bridge may take up to 18 months.
8. Once the bridge has formed the canal may be obturated using a warm vertical condensation technique with gutta percha or use of a thermoplasticised gutta percha delivery system.

There is some evidence that prolonged use of calcium hydroxide in root canals weakens the dentine and therefore apexification with calcium hydroxide should not be the first choice of treatment in these cases.

Create apical barrier with MTA

Mineral trioxide aggregate (MTA) has been used successfully to create a barrier at the apex of open-apex incisors. Rather than using the apexification technique above, MTA should be used to create a barrier at the apex to allow obturation with gutta percha in the remainder of the canal (Fig. 31.2). It is not recommended that MTA is placed through the whole length of the canal. It is also not recommended that MTA be used in teeth that are undergoing replacement resorption as it will be very difficult to remove the material from the bone once the tooth is gone. The technique is as follows:

1. Clean root canal and dress with calcium hydroxide paste for at least 1 week.
2. Mix MTA immediately before its use, powder : sterile water (3 : 1).
3. Carry mix in an MTA applicator.
4. Lightly condense the MTA with pluggers or back end of paper points.
5. Create a 3–4 mm apical plug and check radiographically.
6. Place a moist cotton pellet/paper point and a temporary restoration until following visit before completing obturation. Quick-setting MTA is also available which allows obturation with GP to be carried out in the same visit.

The main advantage of MTA is that it allows the endodontic treatment to be completed over far fewer visits compared with when apexification is induced with calcium hydroxide.

Regenerative endodontic technique (RET)

This relatively new technique (regenerative endodontic technique) has been proposed that aims to debride and sterilise the root canal and then induce bleeding; this allows vital tissue to regenerate and recolonise the root canal with precursor cells that will promote continued root development (Fig. 31.3). The technique involves:

1. Debridement of the canal.
2. Disinfection with a mixture of three antibiotics which are used in the canal for 2–3 weeks:
   ○ metronidazole 20 mg/ml;
   ○ cefachlor 20 mg/ml;
   ○ ciprofloxacin 20 mg/ml.
3. Instrumentation past the apex to promote bleeding within the canal and formation of a blood clot.
4. Placement of a biocompatible material such as Portland cement or another material at the cervical region to seal the canal.
5. Placement of glass ionomer to seal the access cavity.
6. Restoration of the tooth with composite resin.
7. Regular review to check for root development.

The blood clot allows recolonisation of the root canal by progenitor cells which are thought to be located in a stem cell rich area around the apical part of developing roots. This has been termed as stem cells of the apical papilla (SCAP). It has been shown that the entire pulpal vascular complex can be reformed with the continued deposition of dentine and completion of root development and apical closure. While there are increasing data to support this technique, the long-term success of this procedure has yet to be determined. However, nothing is lost if the procedure fails and in the event of failure, an apexification procedure may be performed. The technique is best performed in cases where the prognosis with conventional techniques is thought to be hopeless.

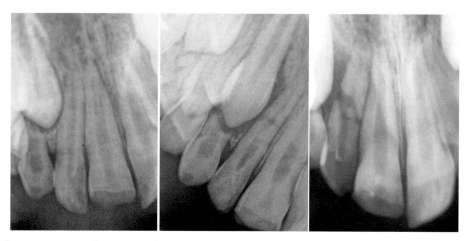

Figure 32.1 When a root fracture is suspected it is essential to take radiographs at different horizontal and vertical angulations. The fracture is not evident on the first radiograph and with elongation, the fracture appears faintly as an ellipse. It is only in the final film that the true extent of the fracture is shown.

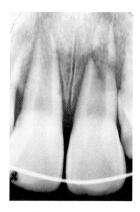

Figure 32.2 High apical root fractures have a very good prognosis especially if the tooth is immature. A rigid stainless steel wire has been used here for splinting.

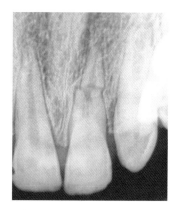

Figure 32.3 A favourable healing outcome of a mid-apical root fracture with continued development of the root fragment and pulp canal obliteration of the coronal segment.

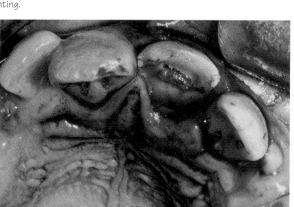

Figure 32.4 A complicated crown/root fracture with the defect extending below the gingival margin and to the level of the crestal bone. In these cases it is important to remove the coronal fragments of the tooth to fully visualise the extent of the fracture and determine whether the tooth is restorable.

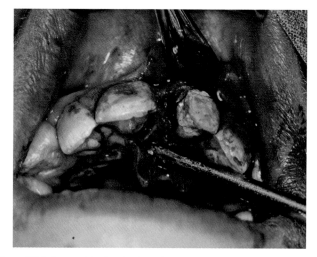

Figure 32.5 Raising labial and palatal flaps to investigate the extent of a complicated crown/root fracture. In this case there is a long vertical fracture. Inevitably, the long-term prognosis is very poor given the difficulty in adequately restoring this defect.

Paediatric Dentistry at a Glance, First Edition. Monty Duggal, Angus Cameron and Jack Toumba. © 2013 John Wiley & Sons Ltd. Published 2013 by Blackwell Publishing Ltd.

Root fractures

Root fractures tend to occur in older children and adolescents. In young children the bone is softer, so teeth tend to be displaced and luxated; however, as the bone becomes harder and teeth more brittle with age, then root fractures are more common.

Diagnosis

• Take several radiographs at different angulations (Fig. 32.1).
• Check for both vertical and horizontal root fractures.
• Fractures may not be evident initially, it is only with inflammation and swelling that the fragments separate and are visible.
• Suspect a vertical root fracture when an isolated periodontal defect is present or there is inability to resolve a periapical infection.
Aim: to align fragments, provide stability and achieve healing.

Management

• Reposition coronal fragment and splint rigidly for up to 12 weeks with composite resin and wire or orthodontic appliances.
• High apical fractures usually require no treatment (Fig. 32.2).
• Review.

Healing

The apical portion of the fracture almost always retains its vitality.
• Hard tissue union between fragments (very uncommon).
• Interposition of bone (Fig. 32.3).
• Interposition of fibrous connective tissue.
• Granulation tissue between fragments – coronal pulp necrosis.

Prognosis

• Depends on height of fracture – the more apical the better the prognosis.
• If close to alveolar crest or with minimal root length, then there is a poor prognosis.

Pulp necrosis of coronal fragment

It is uncommon for the apical fragment to become necrotic. If pulp necrosis of the coronal fragment occurs, there will be radiographic signs of bone loss at the level of the fracture. Other symptoms, such as pain, excessive mobility or gingival swelling and sinus formation, may also be present.
• Extirpate the pulp from coronal fragment only.
• Do not instrument past the fracture line.
• Perform apexification – this may take up to 18 months.
• Obturate up to the barrier, classically or with MTA.

Pulp necrosis of both apical and coronal fragments

• Poor prognosis generally.
• Apicectomy is required to remove apical portion then manage as described above for the coronal fragment.

Crown/root fractures

Initially remove the coronal fragments to determine how far the fracture extends subgingivally.

Uncomplicated crown/root fracture

• Gingivectomy or gingivoplasty to expose margin if required.
• Restore with glass ionomer and composite resin.
• It may not be necessary to fully restore the defect as a long junctional epithelial attachment will form over exposed dentine.

Complicated crown/root fracture (Fig. 32.4)

If the fracture extends below the crestal bone and the root development is complete remove the coronal fragments to assess the extent of the fracture and extirpate the pulp. Calcium hydroxide or Ledermix paste may be placed as the initial endodontic dressing.

If the crown/root fracture does not extend below the crestal bone, and the root development is complete, a Cvek pulpotomy may be performed. This type of fracture may be restorable with glass ionomer over the dentine and composite resin, while deeper fractures usually require advanced prosthodontic options. Unfortunately, the long-term prognosis for such a tooth is not good (Fig. 32.5).

Management

• Similar to a high root fracture.
• Gingivectomy to expose fracture margin. This is usually a better option to allow the defect to be cleaned.
• Cast crowns with extended shoulder, but periodontal surgery may also be required to gain access to the defect for a good impression.
• Orthodontic extrusion of the root to expose the fracture margin. This will allow exposure of the fracture margin but will decrease the crown to root ratio and narrow the emergence profile. It may not provide an acceptable aesthetic result due to the narrow cervical width.
• Root burial or decoronation. Decoronation is essentially a short-term measure that will preserve bone height for later prosthodontic management. Maintenance of the alveolar width may be essential for later implant placement.
• Extraction. In some cases, the tooth may be unrestorable, but the decision to extract should be made following consultation with an orthodontist. With crowding, it may be desirable to close spaces, while in those cases with an excess of space, prosthodontic options may be the only alternative.

Crown/root fractures in immature teeth

These are relatively rare fractures and while immature teeth will have much more potential to heal, their prognosis will depend on the level of the fracture. Invariably, the prognosis is poor for any tooth with a fracture that extends below the gingival margin and also involves the pulp in an immature tooth. As mentioned previously, the apical portion almost always retains its vitality. Treatment planning in these cases should always consider the long-term options and even in hopeless cases, it may be desirable to retain the tooth until growth or dental development has been completed.

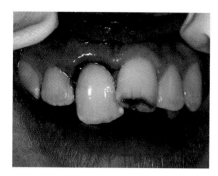

Figure 33.1 Lateral luxation. In most cases there are a combination of injuries. The upper right central incisor has been slightly extruded in addition to a lateral luxation.

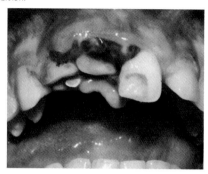

Figure 33.2 Intrusive luxation.

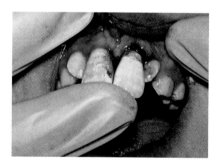

Figure 33.3 Replantation of an avulsed permanent central incisor with finger pressure. Usually the tooth will "click" back into the correct position if replanted early.

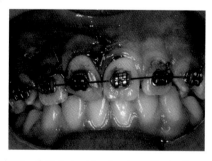

Figure 33.4 Splinting of an avulsed tooth using orthodontic appliances. These have the advantage that they can be placed very quickly and the wire can be removed and replaced as required. There also tends to be less damage to the enamel when removing the brackets compared to using excessive amounts of composite resin.

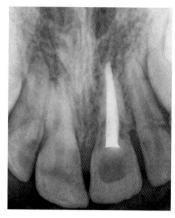

Figure 33.5 Usually avulsed teeth are lost by replacement resorption. Avulsed teeth are a periodontal problem and not an endodontic problem. It is the damage to the periodontal ligament and the death of the supporting cells that results in ankylosis and eventual tooth loss.

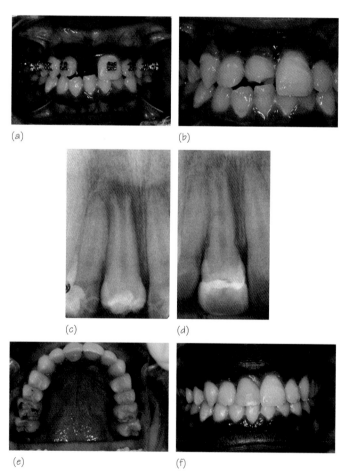

Figure 33.6 (a–f) A completed case showing the use of premolar transplant to upper right central incisor region. Note continued root development of the transplant (d).

Paediatric Dentistry at a Glance, First Edition. Monty Duggal, Angus Cameron and Jack Toumba. © 2013 John Wiley & Sons Ltd. Published 2013 by Blackwell Publishing Ltd.

Concussion and subluxation

These teeth are not displaced and can be managed conservatively and treated symptomatically. They have a good prognosis.
- Splinting is not required.
- Baseline radiographs and pulp tests.

Lateral and extrusive luxation

These teeth need to be repositioned as soon as possible. After 24 hours it is usually very difficult to replace the teeth in the original position (Fig. 33.1).
1. Baseline periapical radiographs.
2. Reposition teeth manually, avoiding any further damage to the root.
3. Non-rigid splinting, although, if multiple teeth are involved, a more rigid wire may be required.
4. Review fortnightly, then at 1, 3, 6 and 12 months.
5. Initial pulp sensibility tests may give false negative readings.
The prognosis for these teeth is usually good, although root canal therapy may be required. Resorption is uncommon, but pulp canal obliteration occurs more frequently in luxated immature teeth. The prognosis is poorer if there is an associated dento-alveolar fracture.

Pulp necrosis in luxated teeth

Teeth need to be monitored for loss of vitality using all available parameters, including radiographic and colour changes. Transient apical breakdown is commonly seen in lateral luxations, but these teeth are not necrotic. Avoid starting root canal treatment unless there are other indicators of infection of the pulp canal.

Intrusion (Fig. 33.2)

The prognosis for most intrusive injuries is poor as the periodontal ligament is crushed against the bone and teeth will usually become ankylosed and lost through replacement resorption.
- If intrusion is minimal and the tooth is only partially erupted then it can be monitored and may re-erupt.
- In all other cases, manually reposition or place orthodontic appliances to extrude the tooth over 7 days and then splint.
- Commence root canal therapy within 10–14 days and place calcium hydroxide as an intra-canal medicament.

Prognosis

- Generally, the prognosis is very poor and almost all teeth will become necrotic.
- If there is progressive resorption, then do not obturate but allow to be replaced by bone.
- Even those teeth that re-erupt spontaneously often undergo pulp necrosis.

Avulsion of permanent teeth

The prognosis of an avulsed tooth is dependent on:
- extra-oral time and storage of the tooth when out of the mouth;
- degree of damage to the root surface.

Management (Figs. 33.3 and 33.4)

1. In spite of the long-term prognosis, all teeth should be replanted immediately if possible. If unable to replant the tooth then store in any available isotonic medium such as: milk, Hank's balanced salt solution, saliva or saline, but DO NOT use water.

2. Give local anaesthesia and debride the tooth socket.
3. Clean the tooth surface gently to remove necrotic debris.
4. Replant teeth with digital pressure until in correct position.
5. Splint with flexible wire or orthodontic brackets for 2 weeks.
6. Antibiotics and tetanus toxoid (if required).

Replanting dry teeth

Teeth that have been out of the mouth for more than 30 minutes may be replanted but will ultimately be lost. While several alternatives have been suggested to minimise replacement resorption, there is little evidence that root scaling, soaking in fluoride, Emdogain® significantly alter outcome. While most of these teeth will be lost, replantation may be beneficial in occlusal development, providing aesthetics in children too young for advanced restorative work and to keep options open for long-term treatment.

Endodontics

It is essential to extirpate within 10 days to avoid the risk of inflammatory root resorption. Inadequately extirpated teeth may resorb within a number of weeks. Alternatively, dry teeth may be extirpated prior to replantation.
- Teeth with very immature roots **may** revascularise if replanted early, but these teeth will **never** respond normally to pulp sensibility tests.

Prognosis

- Periodontal ligament cells will not survive past 30 minutes but may be still viable up to 2 hours when stored in a suitable medium.
- Pulp necrosis occurs in **all** teeth with closed apices.
- Most teeth are lost by replacement resorption (Fig. 33.5).
Factors to consider in treatment planning:
- the long-term prognosis of the tooth, infraoccluding teeth should be decoronated;
- orthodontic considerations;
- loss of bone height and alveolar width;
- the importance of the tooth for arch development;
- social reasons for keeping the tooth.

Autotransplantation

Premolar auto transplantation is a well recognised technique for managing missing anterior teeth, including teeth lost through trauma. Advantages are:
- natural tooth replacement rather than bridge, denture or osseo-integrated implant;
- bone inductive properties;
- normal marginal gingival contour;
- possibility of orthodontic tooth movement;
- treatment in the growing patient.
An early orthodontic opinion is required to identify if extraction of premolars is needed as a part of a future orthodontic plan. If the donor tooth has incomplete root development revascularisation is expected with continued root development. For those teeth with mature root apices, endodontic treatment is commenced within 1 week of transplantation. Careful multidisciplinary treatment planning is the key to success (Fig. 33.6).

34 Diagnosis, biopsy and investigation of pathology in children

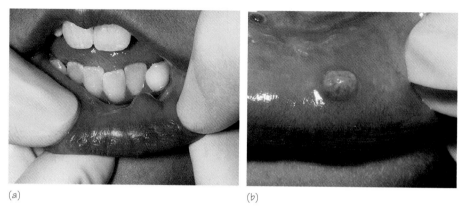

(a)   (b)

Figure 34.1 *Different presentations of a mucocoele. (a) The typical presentation of a painless fluid-filled lesion on the lower lip. (b) This lesion is long standing and is fibrosed and keratotic on the surface.*

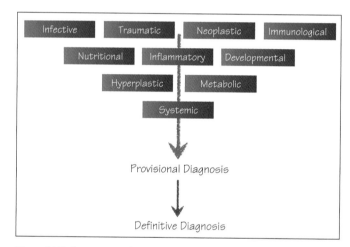

Figure 34.2 *One example of a surgical or diagnostic sieve.*

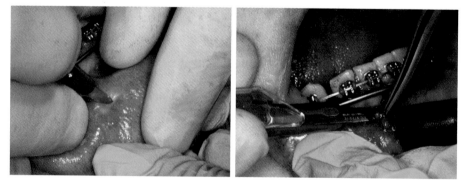

Figure 34.3 *Performing a biopsy of a lesion on the lower lip.*

Paediatric Dentistry at a Glance, First Edition. Monty Duggal, Angus Cameron and Jack Toumba. © 2013 John Wiley & Sons Ltd. Published 2013 by Blackwell Publishing Ltd.

Oral pathology in children

Fortunately, serious pathology in children is rare. Nonetheless, it is essential for the clinician to understand the different nature of presentation of pathology in children, that may be quite different from that which presents in an adult, and that lesions may change over time with growth and development. Generally, the earlier the appearance of pathology the more potentially serious may be the outcome. Oral manifestations may also point to systemic disease and must be fully investigated.

How to diagnose

Diagnosis is like solving a puzzle. Unfortunately, not all the pieces of the puzzle may be present or may have to be found. There must be a logical approach to the diagnosis of any pathological condition. Clinicians must not rely on the mere recognition of a condition from experience, from memory or from a text-book photograph. Pathology may have multiple presentations depending on the stage of the development of the lesion, the age of the patient or possibly on environmental factors (Fig. 34.1). Conversely, one presentation may be representative of any number of different pathological lesions.

Variations of normal must be separated from pathology. While rarities exist and must be excluded, always consider the most likely diagnosis first. The great majority of lesions in children may resolve within a few weeks (such as an ulcer), often without a diagnosis; however, there is great skill in recognising those lesions that are serious and require further investigation and those that can be observed.

Stages in management of pathology

1. Identification and recognition.
2. History and examination.
3. Differential diagnosis.
4. Investigations.
5. Provisional diagnosis.
6. Definitive diagnosis.
7. Treatment and management.

Diagnosis by presentation

How can a clinician hope to remember all the possible conditions that may present in a patient? One method to aid diagnosis is the grouping of conditions by presentation (all conditions presenting with ulceration). As mentioned above, this may be problematic in that some conditions have multiple presentations. However, this book will divide lesions by presentation as this is how the clinician first observes the condition.

The diagnostic or "surgical" sieve and the differential diagnosis (Fig. 34.2)

The diagnostic or surgical sieve may be a more useful tool in the development of a differential diagnosis. It is important to consider all the possible conditions that may be present.

The use of a surgical sieve assists the clinician to consider all different possibilities that may exist. Once a differential diagnosis has been developed this is refined with the aid of other investigations to develop a provisional diagnosis. A definitive diagnosis can only be determined following histopathological examination. While there are many forms of surgical sieve, one should be chosen that covers all possible diagnostic groups and allows the clinician to develop a diagnosis from first principles. Each grouping may be further subdivided, for example an infection may be caused by bacteria, viruses or fungi.

When to investigate

When treating children consideration must be given to the risks of investigations. There may be long-term effects of invasive tests on growing tissues including the effects of radiation, scarring from surgery, interference with growth and development and, of course, the psychological effects of possible surgical treatment. Always consider the child's need for anaesthesia and sedation.

If a lesion has not resolved within 14 days then there is a requirement to investigate further. Rapid changes or deterioration of the condition may also precipitate the need for intervention. If there is a question as to the diagnosis and there has been little or no change, then there is often room for caution and observation. This is often a question of clinical experience.

Investigative tests

Clinicians must be familiar with the full range of tests and investigations appropriate to the presentation of the condition. There is no excuse for "blanket testing". The ordering of any investigation must be carefully considered and be of benefit in diagnosis and management of the condition.

The results of blood tests by themselves do not usually reveal an answer and must be interpreted in relation to all the other information concerning the pathology. Normal ranges are published for each laboratory, however, these may change with the child's age or other events such as infection or growth during puberty.

- Dental investigations.
- Blood tests - haematology, clinical chemistry.
- Radiography and other imaging.
- Microbiology, cytology, histopathology.

Biopsy (Fig. 34.3)

Biopsy and histopathological examination is often the only way in which a definitive diagnosis may be made. The decision to undertake a surgical procedure in a child must be weighed against the possible complications associated with the removal of tissue from potentially sensitive areas. Consideration must also be given to who should perform the surgery. If a malignancy or other serious condition is a possibility, then it is best to refer the child to the clinician who will be responsible for the final management. Always take a representative sample. The centre of the lesion may be ulcerated however this area may not be diagnostic. Other factors include:

- Excisional or incisional biopsy?
- Take a representative tissue sample.
- Include an adequate size of tissue that can be examined with a border of normal tissue.
- Consider adjacent structures.
- Is sedation or general anaesthesia required?
- What histopathological tests are to be ordered?

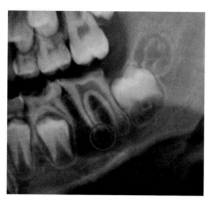

Figure 35.1 Periapical area associated with a necrotic lower first permanent molar.

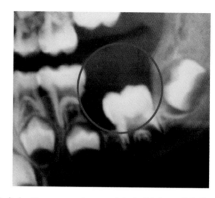

Figure 35.2 A dentigerous cyst associated with lower left first permanent molar that has resorbed the roots of the second primary molar.

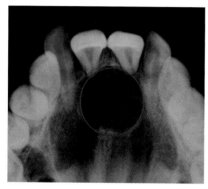

Figure 35.3 Incisive canal cyst: a single, isolated lesion in the palate not associated with the dentition.

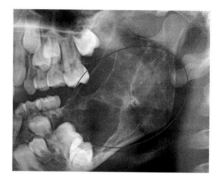

Figure 35.4 The ramus of mandible in a child with cherubism showing the typical "soap-bubble" appearance.

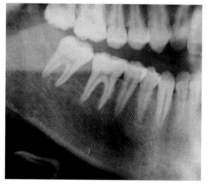

Figure 35.5 Generalised bony rarefaction and diffuse bony changes in the trabecular pattern in a child with a metastatic fibrosarcoma from the abdomen.

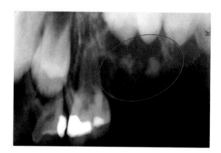

Figure 35.6 A mixed lesion with radio-opacities inside a radiolucent lesion typical of ameloblastic fibro-odontoma.

Box 35.1 Periapical radiolucencies

Periapical granuloma, surgical defect
Radicular cyst
Traumatic bone cyst

Box 35.2 Radiolucencies associated with the crowns of unerupted teeth

Dentigerous (follicular) cyst
Inflammatory follicular cyst
Eruption cyst
Ameloblastic fibroma
Ameloblastic fibro-odontoma
Ossifying fibroma
Odontogenic keratocyst

Paediatric Dentistry at a Glance, First Edition. Monty Duggal, Angus Cameron and Jack Toumba. © 2013 John Wiley & Sons Ltd. Published 2013 by Blackwell Publishing Ltd.

Box 35.3 Separate isolated radiolucencies

Primordial cyst
Traumatic bone cyst
Odontogenic keratocyst
Aneurysmal bone cyst
Fissural cyst
Median palatine cyst
Incisive canal cyst
Central giant cell granuloma
Ossifying fibroma
Hyperparathyroidism

Box 35.4 Multiple or multilocular radiolucencies

Central giant cell tumour
Cherubism (familial fibrous dysplasia)
Langerhans' cell histiocytosis
Odontogenic myxoma
Other metastatic or invasive neoplasms
Central vascular lesion, arteriovenous malformation

Box 35.5 Generalised bony rarefactions

Hyperparathyroidism
Thalassaemia
Langerhans' cell histiocytosis
Fibrous dysplasia
Osteopetrosis

Box 35.6 Mixed lesions with radio-opacities and radiolucencies

Odontoma
Ameloblastic fibro-odontoma
Calcifying odontogenic cyst
Odontogenic fibroma
Adenomatoid odontogenic tumour
Fibrous dysplasia
Ossifying fibroma
Garré's osteomyelitis

Guides to diagnosis

Examination of the radiographic appearance of a particular lesion will aid in the development of a differential diagnosis. Consider the:

- location of the lesion;
- association with other anatomic structures;
- definition of margins;
- internal nature of the lesion.

Is the lesion rapidly expanding where there is resorption of adjacent structures or is it slowly growing with associated soft tissue expansion and movement of the teeth? The possible diagnoses listed below are representative of pathology found in children and are not meant to be all inclusive.

Periapical radiolucencies (Fig. 35.1 and Box 35.1)

The majority of these lesions are associated with the loss of vitality of a tooth. While a tooth may have been treated with root canal therapy, a residual defect or healing area may remain for many months and the isolated presence of a periapical area may not necessarily indicate ongoing pathology.

Radiolucencies associated with the crowns of unerupted teeth (Fig. 35.2 and Box 35.2)

These lesions are odontogenic and are related to changes in the follicle around the developing tooth. Associated teeth tend to be displaced away from the lesion and consequently away from the occlusal plane. Cysts associated with mandibular teeth commonly result in migration of those teeth inferiorly and posteriorly, while in the maxilla, the teeth move superiorly and inferiorly.

Separate isolated radiolucencies (Fig. 35.3 and Box 35.3)

Separate isolated radiolucencies tend to be non-odontogenic. The location may assist in the diagnosis and many are developmental or associated with systemic pathology.

Multiple or multilocular radiolucencies (Fig. 35.4 and Box 35.4)

The appearance of a multiloculated lesion in the jaws must always be regarded with concern. They are uncommon but mostly associated with a neoplasm or systemic illness.

Generalised bony rarefactions (Fig. 35.5 and Box 35.5)

Polyostotic, generalised or diffuse changes in the bone of the jaws are invariably associated with systemic or metabolic disease. Some of these conditions may have multiple presentations, such as hyperparathyroidism that may present with separate isolated radiolucencies (Brown's tumours of bone) or in a more generalised way with more generalised bone density loss.

Mixed lesions with radio-opacities and radiolucencies (Fig. 35.6 and Box 35.6)

A mixed lesion may present initially as an isolated radiopacity which over time develops a mixed appearance with islands of calcification.

Radio-opacities in the jaws

Isolated radio-opacities in the jaws are related to highly calcified areas or foreign bodies that may appear to be solely radio-opaque or mixed, in early stages prior to undergoing calcification. Again, these lesions may be radiolucent or mixed initially before undergoing calcification.

36 Management of odontogenic infections in children

Table 36.1 Common antibiotic dosages for children.

Antibiotic	Dosage	Frequency	Administration	Notes
Amoxicillin	15–25 mg/kg	3× daily	Oral	Excellent broad spectrum, active against most oral flora
Penicillin VK	10–12.5 mg/kg	4× daily	Oral	Not to be given with food
Cephalexin	12.5–25 mg/kg	4× daily	Oral	First-generation cephalosporin, second choice after amoxicillin
Benzylpenicillin	30 mg/kg	3× daily	IV	First choice when IV administration is needed
Metronidazole	10 mg/kg	2× daily	Oral	Active against Gram-negative organisms, for severe infections
Clindamycin	10 mg/kg	3× daily	Oral or IV	For those children with an allergy to penicillin

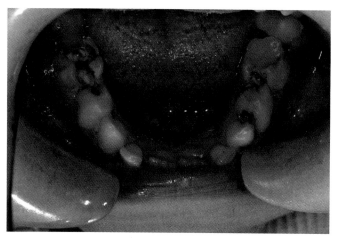

Figure 36.1 A child with mixed dentition with multiple chronic abscesses associated with carious primary teeth. Infection such as this involving primary teeth cannot be treated by pulp therapy. These teeth require extraction.

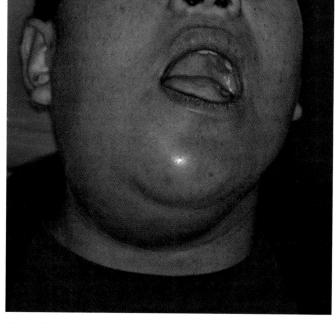

Figure 36.2 A severe and acute submandibular odontogenic infection that requires immediate attention. Any floor-of-mouth swelling or a swelling causing dysphagia or respiratory obstruction is potentially life threatening.

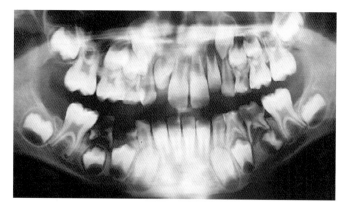

Figure 36.3 A gum-boil is a localised infection that does not require antibiotics. It is more important to treat the cause of the infection and extract the tooth or extirpate the pulp.

Paediatric Dentistry at a Glance, First Edition. Monty Duggal, Angus Cameron and Jack Toumba. © 2013 John Wiley & Sons Ltd. Published 2013 by Blackwell Publishing Ltd.

Odontogenic infections

Infections in the head and neck are serious and must be treated with consideration of the risk of spread. Bacterial infections of the face can be life threatening if inappropriately treated. Children will usually present much earlier than adults and it is important to remember that such infections in young children will progress more rapidly than in adults, but similarly, once managed appropriately, will also resolve faster.

Principles of care

1. Removal of the cause of the infection:
   ○ extraction;
   ○ pulpectomy.
2. Surgical drainage if required.
3. Antibiotics (Table 36.1).
4. Maintenance of fluid balance.
5. Pain control.

History and presentation

Children usually present early with acute infection that is most commonly a cellulitis rather than an abscess and a frank collection of pus. The child may be febrile and acutely unwell and there would usually be a history of previous toothache. Following several days of pain, a swelling may arise overnight with a relief of pain. This is due to the infection breaching the cortical plate of bone and then spreading through fascial planes. Lymph nodes may be enlarged.

Organisms involved and antibiotics

Typical odontogenic infections in children present with mixed flora that are principally Gram-positive facultative anaerobes including streptococci, *Fusobacterium* and *Bacteroides* subspecies. In this regard, it is important to choose an antibiotic that has a broad spectrum with activity against these organisms. Fortunately most oral organisms are sensitive to the synthetic penicillins and amoxicillin, or a first-generation cephalosporin should be the drug of first choice. Erythromycin is generally bacteriostatic and a gastric irritant in children and for those children with sensitivity to penicillins, clindamycin is a better alternative. For those children with severe orofacial infections, the addition of metronidazole may be appropriate.

Spread of infection

Note the location and spread of the infection and swelling. Maxillary swellings originate in the canine fossa and spread superiorly to involve the infraorbital region. In severe cases there may be posterior spread with cavernous sinus thrombosis and brain abscess. The spread of infections of mandibular teeth will be determined by the relation of the roots to the mylohyoid muscle sling. Primary teeth, whose roots lie above the mylohyoid, usually involve the buccal vestibule then spread inferiorly to the submandibular area. An abscess arising from the lower first permanent molar may present with a floor of mouth swelling involving the submandibular, submental and sublingual tissue spaces. Any collection of pus in these areas requires surgical drainage. Ludwig's angina is an uncommon presentation in young children but any swelling involving the floor of the mouth or one that crosses the midline must be managed aggressively to avoid possible airway obstruction or further inferior spread to the mediastinum.

Treat the cause of the problem

Always treat the cause of the infection. While the prescription of antibiotics will aid in the management of the acute infection, they are not a substitute for removing the cause, namely extraction or pulp extirpation. In cases where a facial swelling is present, extraction of the offending primary tooth is indicated.

Extraction vs pulp extirpation (Fig. 36.1)

Infections or significant collections of pus arising from necrotic primary teeth cannot be drained through the tooth roots alone and these teeth require removal. Abscessed permanent molars may be treated with root canal therapy although the long-term prognosis of a grossly carious tooth should be considered in a young child.

Pain control and anaesthesia

It may be difficult to achieve adequate local anaesthesia to allow extraction in the presence of acute inflammation. The use of relative analgesia or other pharmacological behaviour management techniques would aid in what is an upsetting and traumatic experience for a young child. Many children with severe swellings will require management under general anaesthesia at which point the teeth can be extracted and drainage achieved. It is important to assess the severity of the infection and the urgency of care.

The need for hospital admission (Fig. 36.2)

Children become unwell and deteriorate quickly. As a general rule, admission should be considered for those children presenting with a temperature above 39 °C or a persistent spiking temperature. Always consider the state of hydration of the child as they may not have eaten or drunk any fluids for some time.

Surgical drainage

Unlike adults, children may not present with significant collections of pus and do not require traditional surgical drainage. However, any pus must be removed. Surgical drains are rarely required, the only exception being those children with very severe submandibular swellings requiring an extra-oral through-and-through drain.

The local dental abscess (Fig. 36.3)

The gum-boil or buccal sinus is a localised abscess and the main tenet remains to remove the cause of the infection by pulp extirpation and pulpectomy or extraction. Antibiotics should not be administered unless there is systemic involvement.

Other diagnoses to consider

- Periorbital cellulitis.
- Actinomycosis.
- Osteomyelitis.
- Atypical mycobacterial infection.
- Salivary gland infections.
- Non-odontogenic infections of the head and neck.

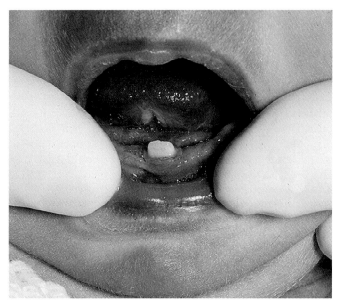

Figure 37.1 *A traumatic ulcer in an infant on the ventral surface of the tongue. This is termed Riga-Fedé ulceration and is often seen in children with cerebral palsy and is caused by rubbing of the tongue over the newly erupted lower incisors.*

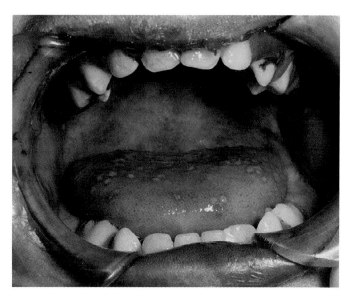

Figure 37.3 *Oral ulceration in primary herpetic gingivostomatitis. It is uncommon to observe the vesicles that rapidly break down to form multiple ulcers that may coalesce. The child is often very unwell and will not tolerate oral fluids or solids.*

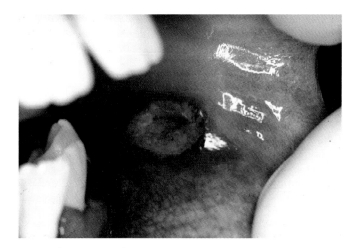

Figure 37.2 *A deep painful ulcer in an immunocompromised child. Any ulcer that does not heal within 2 weeks requires further investigation.*

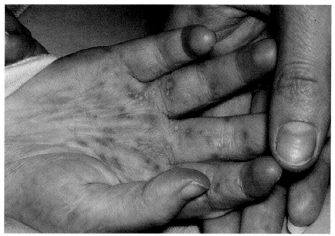

Figure 37.4 *The typical target lesions on the hand of a child suffering erythema multiforme. The child also has a panoral stomatitis with much of the oral mucosa ulcerating and forming a slough. Debridement of the oral cavity and removal of the necrotic debris is very important.*

Paediatric Dentistry at a Glance, First Edition. Monty Duggal, Angus Cameron and Jack Toumba. © 2013 John Wiley & Sons Ltd. Published 2013 by Blackwell Publishing Ltd.

Diagnosis

Ulceration is a non-specific sign of full-thickness epithelial breakdown. It may occur as a result of trauma (Fig. 37.1), such as biting the lip following an inferior alveolar nerve block injection, viral infection or immunological disease (Fig. 37.2), including any of the conditions mentioned later. Any ulcerative lesion in a child that fails to resolve within 2 weeks requires further investigation. While the aetiology of most ulcers may be determined by history and examination, long-standing or recurrent ulceration in children often requires investigative blood tests and possibly biopsy. Blood investigations might include:
* full blood count with differential white cell count;
* electrolytes;
* iron studies including ferritin, red cell folate and total iron-binding capacity;
* serum vitamin B_{12};
* anti-nuclear antibodies;
* anti-gliadin antibodies;
* serum angiotensin converting enzyme (ACE);
* C-reactive protein.

Management of oral ulceration

In most cases the management is symptomatic and empirical but treatment of any underlying nutritional or haematological deficiency is paramount. Topical antiseptics and steroids give some relief and, in severe cases, systemic steroids may be required:
* mouthrinses:
  ◦ 0.2% chlorhexidine gluconate;
  ◦ 1.2% benzydamine hydrochloride;
* sulfasalazine;
* topical steroids:
  ◦ triamcinolone in Orabase.

Viral infections of childhood

Any viral infections may present with an intraoral involvement. Commonly, these are seasonal or epidemic making the diagnosis easier. All present with a characteristic prodrome of 24–48 hours of febrile illness of varying severity followed by the appearance of vesicles that breakdown rapidly to form painful small ulcers. These may coalesce and result in large areas of ulceration. Children with severe oral ulceration may be in great distress and unable to eat or drink, complicating their management.

Primary herpetic gingivostomatitis (Fig. 37.3)

Primary herpes is the most common cause of a young child presenting with oral ulceration, although while 70% of adults have been exposed to the herpes simplex virus (HSV) less than 1% have a severe primary infection. Oral herpes typically results from type I infection, however, type II may also infect the oral cavity and they are clinically indistinguishable. Primary herpes is almost unknown prior to the eruption of teeth but may present coincidentally with the first emergence of teeth and a breach of the oral epithelium. Vesicles appear anywhere in the mouth and there is often an intense inflammation of the gingival tissues with or without ulceration. The child may be very unwell and febrile with a marked halitosis.

Diagnosis

The diagnosis is usually clinical based on the presentation and the history of exposure to a family member or acquaintance with cold sores, although exfoliative cytology and viral culturing is available.

Management

While primary herpes is a self-limiting disease within about 10 days, young children may become dehydrated quickly, requiring fluid maintenance. Much of the pain from oral ulceration results from secondary bacterial infection and good debridement with oral antiseptics such as 0.2% chlorhexidine gluconate can be of great benefit. Adequate use of analgesics, such as paracetamol, is also required. Children should be encouraged to drink as much as possible. In severe cases, antivirals such as acyclovir may be required.

Coxsackie group A infections

Herpangina and hand, foot and mouth disease are caused by epidemic outbreaks of coxsackie viruses. They present with similar but less severe prodromes and the ulceration is usually limited to the pharynx, the soft palate and the fauces. Obviously, in the latter disease, ulceration with an erythematous border is also present on the palmar and plantar surfaces. Both are self-limiting infections and care is symptomatic, similar to that of primary herpes.

Other viral infections

Other viral infections that may also cause oral ulceration include:
* Epstein–Barr infection presenting as infectious mononucleosis;
* varicella – chickenpox;
* cytomegalovirus.

Vesiculobullous lesions

There are a number of autoimmune diseases that may present with ulceration or intra- or sub-epithelial vesicles or bullae that breakdown resulting in ulceration.

Recurrent minor aphthous ulceration

RAU is relatively common in children affecting perhaps up to 20% of the population. Crops of up to six small, shallow, painful ulcers appear regularly and heal without scarring. The cause is unknown, but usually disappears by middle-age.

Erythema multiforme and Stevens–Johnson syndrome

These conditions present with a panoral stomatitis that appears to be initiated by reactivation of HSV infection, *Mycoplasma* infection or a drug reaction. Erythema multiforme (Fig. 37.4) presents with characteristic target lesions on the palms of the hands, while Stevens–Johnson syndrome has genital and ocular involvement.

Other immunological diseases

* Beçhet's syndrome.
* Pemphigus.
* Lupus erythematosus.
* Orofacial granulomatosis.
* Crohn disease.

Swellings and enlargements of the gingiva

Box 38.1 Differential diagnosis of gingival swellings

Fibrous epulis
Pyogenic granuloma
Peripheral giant cell granuloma
Squamous papilloma/viral warts
Granular cell tumour of infancy – congenital epulis
Condyloma acuminatum
Eruption cyst
Mucocoele
Lymphangioma
Tuberous sclerosis

Table 38.1 Drugs associated with gingival enlargement.

Drugs associated with gingival enlargement		Alternatives
Anticonvulsants	Phenytoin	Tegretol
Immunosuppressives	Cyclosporin	Tacrolimus
	Azathioprine?	
Calcium channel blockers	Nifedipine	
	Diltiazem	
	Verapamil	

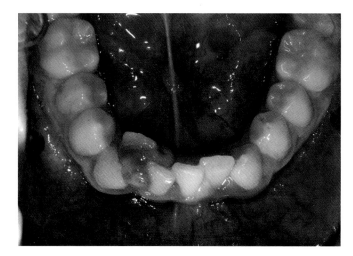

Figure 38.1 A gingival epulis. Most of these lesions are reactive and represent an overgrowth of tissue in response to mild irritation. Surgical removal is straightforward but must include a border of normal tissue. Most do not recur.

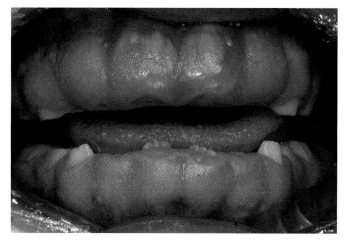

Figure 38.2 Gingival enlargement in a child with hereditary gingival fibromatosis. The teeth have been almost totally obscured and surgical resection is required. There is very little inflammation and the overgrowth is not related to plaque or oral hygiene.

Paediatric Dentistry at a Glance, First Edition. Monty Duggal, Angus Cameron and Jack Toumba. © 2013 John Wiley & Sons Ltd. Published 2013 by Blackwell Publishing Ltd.

Epulides (Box 38.1)

An epulis is a swelling on the gingiva and is a non-specific term. Most epulides are inflammatory or reactive lesions to plaque or other gingival irritants. They are usually well circumscribed and pedunculated and, while the precise cause may not be determined, they are easily managed by surgical excision with a small border of normal tissue. It is important to remember that some of these lesions have a large vascular component and may bleed excessively on removal.

Pyogenic granuloma/fibrous epulis (Fig. 38.1)

Perhaps the most common epulis, the misnamed pyogenic granuloma (no pus is present) is a slow-growing, well circumscribed, usually pedunculated lesion that is a more highly vascular variant of the fibrous epulis. They are extremely variable in appearance and usually arise from the inderdental papilla. Some authors describe this as a form of capillary haemangioma.

Peripheral giant cell granuloma

This lesion occurs only in the region of the primary dentition and is usually dark in colour. Importantly they have a tendency to regrow if not completely excised. There is a characteristic radiographic cupping of the bone and histologically they have numerous multinucleated giant cells.

Papilloma/viral warts/condyloma acuminatum

Most papillomas and viral warts in children are associated with the human papilloma virus and are verrucous exophytic growths. They are commonly associated with extra-oral lesions on the hands and feet. Condyloma acuminatum may be of similar appearance and its presence may require investigation of possible sexual assault, as this lesion is usually considered to be a venereal disease.

Eruption cyst

Eruption cysts are merely enlargements of the dental follicle that appear just prior to tooth eruption. They may be bluish in appearance and may mimic a vascular lesion and it is important to exclude the possibility that the lesion will bleed profusely. Rarely do they require any treatment other than reassurance and teeth erupt normally through the cyst. It is uncommon that these lesions become infected.

Tuberous sclerosis

Children affected with tuberous sclerosis suffer from epilepsy and an intellectual disability. They also have a pitting hypoplasia of the enamel, characteristically on the labial surface of the incisors, and vascular epulides on their gingivae. Being angiomas, they may bleed excessively during removal.

Congenital epulis

This lesion is present at birth and is also termed a granular cell tumour of infancy (see Chapter 39).

Peripheral ossifying fibroma

This lesion is very similar in appearance to a pyogenic granuloma; it is reactive in nature and is characterised by a fibrous connective tissue stroma intermingled with islands of dystrophic calcification.

Management

All lesions should be conservatively excised with a border of normal tissue. Maintenance of oral hygiene is essential if many of these lesions are not to recur. Be aware that some lesions are highly vascular. The final diagnosis is almost always determined by histopathological examination and all excised tissue should be sent for examination by a pathologist.

Gingival enlargements

Generalised gingival enlargements or overgrowths may be reactive to plaque, drug-induced (Table 38.1) or hereditary.

Pathogenesis:
- plaque-induced gingival enlargement;
- connective tissue enlargement;
- increase in extracellular protein matrix;
- fibrogenic response to drug;
- ? decreased collagen degradation.

Phenytoin (Dilantin) enlargement

Enlargement of the interdental papilla is characteristic of phenytoin enlargement. While there appears to be a dose-related response, the role of plaque control is extremely important and if plaque control cannot be maintained then regrowth will occur.

Cyclosporin A enlargement

While a number of newer immunosuppressive drugs exist that do not cause gingival overgrowth such as tacrolimus, cyclosporin remains the main drug of choice following organ transplantation. The side affects of gingival overgrowth appear not to be dose related and not all children will suffer this condition. However, a number of children are also administered calcium channel blockers such as nifedipine and verapamil to control hypertension post transplantation and both are also associated with gingival enlargement.

Hereditary gingival fibromatosis (Fig. 38.2)

There are a number of syndromes associated with gingival overgrowth or enlargement. Hereditary gingival fibromatosis is an autosomal dominant condition where all the gingival tissues are affected in both arches. Commonly, the primary teeth are delayed in exfoliation and there may be ectopic or delayed eruption of the permanent teeth. The growth of the gingivae may be quite extensive. These differ from the drug-induced overgrowth in that the enlargement is independent of plaque. Repeated surgical resection is usually required but this needs careful treatment planning and timing so as to facilitate the emergence of the permanent teeth.

Management

In all cases, there should be a consideration of the concerns of the child and parent in regard to the appearance of the mouth and the need for repeated surgery to remove excessive gingival tissue.
- Meticulous oral hygiene.
- Gingivectomy or periodontal flap procedure to recontour and allow eruption of teeth.

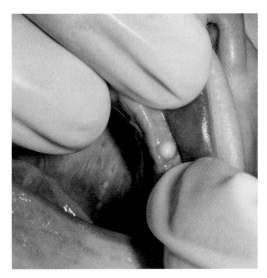

Figure 39.1 A single large Bohn nodule in a neonate. Commonly, multiple lesions are present and vanish within a few months.

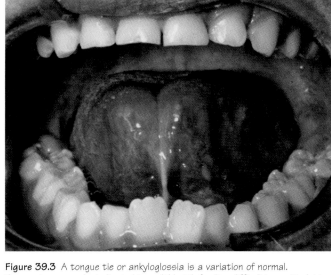

Figure 39.3 A tongue tie or ankyloglossia is a variation of normal. Fraenectomy may be indicated in a child with feeding difficulties, articulation disorders or trauma to the lingual periodontal tissues.

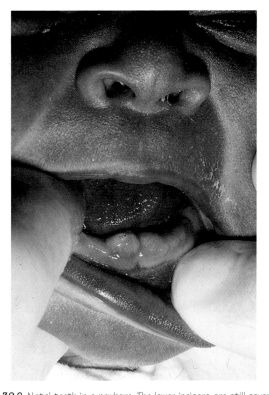

Figure 39.2 Natal teeth in a newborn. The lower incisors are still covered by the follicle. The teeth that will emerge shortly are the normal primary incisors, however, only 5/6ths of the crown will be formed. Only excessively mobile teeth require removal.

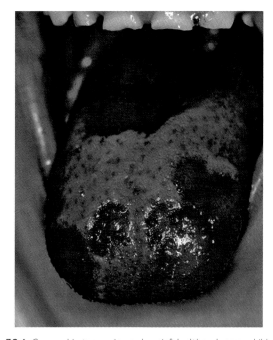

Figure 39.4 Geographic tongue is rarely painful, although some children complain of sensitivity when eating spicy or salty foods due to the erosion and loss of epithelium.

Paediatric Dentistry at a Glance, First Edition. Monty Duggal, Angus Cameron and Jack Toumba. © 2013 John Wiley & Sons Ltd. Published 2013 by Blackwell Publishing Ltd.

Serious oral pathology in newborns and young infants is fortunately very uncommon and many of the "abnormalities" that are observed by the parent or our medical and nursing colleagues are in fact variations of normal. With the advent of more specialised antenatal ultrasound imaging techniques, many congenital abnormalities such as clefts of the lip and palate and cardiac defects can be detected *in utero*.

Developmental cysts of newborns

Epstein's pearls

It is estimated Epstein's pearls may be found in up to 80% of all newborns. These small pale white well circumscribed papules appear in the midline of the palate, usually at the junction of the hard and soft palates, and are true keratinised cysts that have arisen from epithelial cells left in areas along the lines of fusion of the palatal shelves. They are sometimes termed inclusion cysts. Over time they sequestrate and resolve without any intervention.

Bohn's nodules (Fig. 39.1)

Similar to Epstein's pearls, these pale white or yellow papules measuring 1–4 mm in size are sometimes termed dental lamina cysts. They are remnants of the dental epithelium that form keratinised cysts and usually occur anywhere on the alveolar ridges, although they are observed predominately on the maxillary arches. They resolve spontaneously.

Granular cell tumours

Two neoplasms present in newborns and infants that are histologically identical. The granular cell tumour of infancy, sometimes termed the congenital epulis or Neumann tumour, is an uncommon lesion that arises from the alveolar processes of either arch. The granular cell myoblastoma is found predominately on the tongue in older individuals.

Congenital epulis

Unlike the granular cell myoblastoma, this lesion is negative for S100 stain. Over 85% of the lesions are found in girls and in many cases, small lesions resolve spontaneously. Only large lesions require treatment and, as they are usually pedunculated, surgical excision is a straightforward procedure. While this is usually an innocuous condition, the authors have observed lesions up to 4 cm in diameter that may interfere with feeding or result in respiratory obstruction.

Natal and neonatal teeth (Fig. 39.2)

Invariably, teeth that are present at birth (natal) or those that erupt soon after birth (neonatal) are merely normal primary teeth that have emerged early and are not supernumerary teeth. Therefore, these teeth are almost always mobile due to lack of root (and crown) development. The early appearance of primary incisors is not associated with any other pathology; however, premature emergence of primary posterior teeth (less than 6 months of age) is usually of concern and should be investigated.

Management

While there are apocryphal stories concerning the risks of an infant aspirating a natal tooth, there is little evidence that these teeth cause much problem for the newborn or the mother. Similarly, it is uncommon that these teeth cause problems with breast-feeding although ulceration of the ventral surface of the tongue may occur.
- If there is excessive mobility then the tooth should be removed.
- The permanent tooth will develop and erupt normally.
- The parents should be advised that this is a true primary incisor.

Abnormalities of the tongue

A number of abnormalities of the tongue present that are regarded as variations of normal anatomy and are usually congenital.

Ankyloglossia (Fig. 39.3)

A tongue-tie is the most common abnormality of the tongue. While there is no pathology associated with this condition, it may interfere with infant feeding, result in disorders of articulation and, in very severe cases, failure to thrive. A fraenectomy may be indicated if:
- there is severe limitation of movement that results in feeding issues or failure to thrive;
- the mother wishes to continue breastfeeding and there are problems with attachment, nipple damage or recurrent mastitis;
- there are articulation errors with interdental production of sounds particularly with /l/, /t/ and /n/;
- there is an insertion of the fraenum into the free gingival margin lingual to the lower incisors resulting in a periodontal defect.

An assessment by a speech pathologist or a lactation consultant is always advisable in relation to feeding and speech problems prior to any intervention.

Macroglossia

True macroglossia is only associated with Beckwith–Wiedemann syndrome, although a number of diseases such as lymphangioma, cystic hygroma or a metabolic storage disease such as the mucopolysaccharidoses may result in enlargement of the tongue due to growth of a lesion within the tongue. Children with trisomy 21 (Down syndrome) do not have macroglossia, however, the tongue appears to be large because it is protruded and often held forward in the mouth.

Geographic tongue (erythema migrans) (Fig. 39.4)

This is found in about 2% of the population and is probably hereditary. Red areas of erosion or desquamation and loss of the filliform papillae appear over time as patches on the ventral surface of the tongue surrounded by white areas. The condition is usually painless and no treatment is required.

Riga-Fedé ulceration

This ulceration may result from trauma to the ventral surface of the tongue following eruption of lower primary incisors. It is commonly found in children with cerebral palsy. Treatment is confined to smoothing of the incisal edges but extraction of the teeth might be necessary in very severe cases.

Table 40.1 Periodontal diseases in children.

Old terminology	Current terminology
Pre-pubertal periodontitis	Generalised aggressive periodontitis
	Periodontitis associated with systemic disease
Localised juvenile periodontitis	Localised aggressive periodontitis
Acute necrotising ulcerative gingivitis (ANUG)	Necrotising periodontal disease

A summary of the proceedings from the meeting that ratified the new nomenclature can be found in Research, Science and Therapy Committee, American Academy of Periodontology (2003).

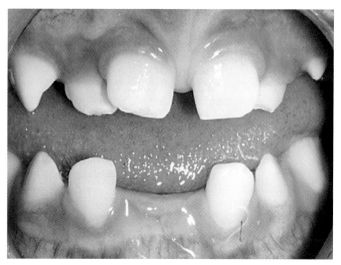

Figure 40.2 Hypophosphatasia due to a deficiency of serum alkaline phosphatase. Note that there is no gingival inflammation and the teeth are not lost due to periodontal disease. There is a lack of cellular cementum in these teeth. Fortunately, only the anterior teeth were lost in this child.

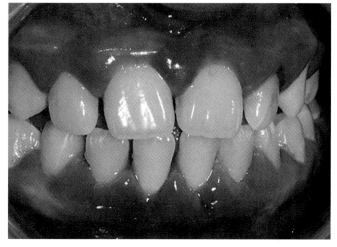

Figure 40.1 Periodontal disease in the primary dentition is extremely rare and always associated with systemic pathology or immune deficiency. There may be little subgingival calculus but note the inflamed gingival tissues and in this case the pocket depth was 5 mm. This child had a deficiency of neutrophils and exfoliated most of her primary teeth over the following 2 years.

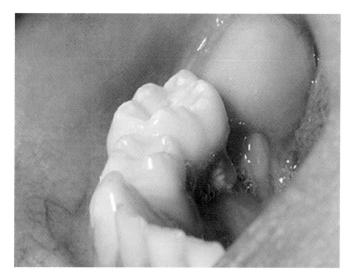

Figure 40.3 Langerhans' cell histiocytosis. The lower second primary molar has almost exfoliated due to bone destruction associated with an eosinophilic granuloma. This child had lesions in all four quadrants.

Paediatric Dentistry at a Glance, First Edition. Monty Duggal, Angus Cameron and Jack Toumba. © 2013 John Wiley & Sons Ltd. Published 2013 by Blackwell Publishing Ltd.

Premature loss of primary teeth

The early exfoliation of primary teeth is invariably associated with serious systemic conditions and requires investigation. Most of these conditions are rare, however, clinicians need to be aware of the uncommon presentation of tooth loss. Early loss of primary teeth can be divided into:
- periodontal disease (Table 40.1);
- metabolic diseases;
- connective tissue disorders;
- neoplasia;
- self-inflicted trauma.

Periodontal disease in children

Gingivitis is common in children but periodontal disease with loss of alveolar bone is rare prior to adolescence and almost always results from a primary immunological disturbance. These may be:
- neutropenias (<1500 cells/ml):
  - congenital neutropenia (Fig. 40.1);
  - cyclic neutropenia;
  - agranulocytosis;
  - neutropenia secondary to chemotherapy;
- qualitative neutrophil disorders (chemotactic or phagocytic defects):
  - leucocyte adhesion defect;
  - Papillon–Lefèvre syndrome;
  - Chédiak–Higashi disease;
  - acatalasia.

Periodontal disease in children is associated with characteristic bacterial flora. These bacteria secrete leucotoxins but they are usually only present in a patient with some form of immunosuppression specifically related to humoral immunity (neutropenia or decreased neutrophil function). B cell defects do not manifest orally but reduced T cell counts usually are associated with periodontal disease and candidiasis.

Characteristic organisms
- *Actinobacillus actinomycetemcomitans.*
- *Provetella intermedia.*
- *Capnocytophaga sputigena.*
- *Eikenelle corrodens.*

Management

The only effective treatment is correction of the immune disorder. The aim must be to try to preserve permanent teeth and this may necessitate extraction of any remaining primary teeth prior to eruption of the permanent teeth. Intensive preventive strategies with antimicrobials, antibiotics and prophylaxis may assist but inevitably most teeth are lost. The prognosis for most children with a severe immunological deficiency is poor and many will die from infection. Bone marrow transplantation (BMT) may be effective in some cases.

Metabolic and connective tissue disorders

These include:
- hypophosphatasia (Fig. 40.2);
- Ehlers–Danlos syndrome (types IV and VIII);

- erythromelalgia;
- arodynia (pink disease from mercury toxicity);
- scurvy.

Hypophosphatasia

This is a rare condition characterised by reduced levels of serum alkaline phosphatase. There appears to be an absence of cellular cementum that results in exfoliation of the teeth in the absence of any periodontal disease.

Diagnosis:
- serum alkaline phosphatase <90 U/l;
- elevated urinary phosphoethanolamine (PEA);
- decreased serum pyridoxal-5-phosphate (vitamin B6);
- bone density scans if required.

Connective tissue disorders

Children with inborn errors in the metabolism of collagen present with hyperextensibility of joints and skin and often bruising and prolonged bleeding due to capillary fragility. Teeth are lost from progressive periodontal disease and loss of attachment.

Neoplasia

- Langerhans' cell histiocytosis (Fig. 40.3).
- Acute myeloid leukaemia.

Langerhans' cell histiocytosis derives from a proliferation of Langerhans' cells. Isolated lesions in the mouth are termed eosinophilic granulomas and may occur in all four quadrants. There is a characteristic appearance of the teeth "floating in air". Other signs include:
- malaise, irritability;
- anogenital and post-auricular rash;
- diabetes insipidus.

Disseminated forms tend to occur in younger children but the overall prognosis of this disease is now good.

Self-injury

- Hereditary sensory neuropathies.
- Lesch–Nyhan syndrome.
- Psychotic or psychological disorders.

All of these conditions are extremely difficult to diagnose initially because of the uncommon and peculiar presentation and they are equally difficult to manage. In the absence of any pathology following routine investigation for the other conditions mentioned above, self-injury must always be included in a differential diagnosis. In some cases the injury may be caused by a close carer (Münchausen's syndrome by proxy).

Management

- Grinding of teeth or composite build-ups to prevent soft tissue damage.
- Acrylic splints or mouthguards.
- In severe cases, extraction of the teeth may be the only alternative.

Missing teeth and extra teeth

Table 41.1 *Stages of tooth development.*

Stage	Appearance	Activity	Examples of disorders
Initiation	Bud stage	Migration of neural crest cells into arches	Hypodontia or supernumerary teeth
Proliferation	Cap stage	Condensation of ectoderm and formation of dental organ and dental papilla	Odontogenic cysts
Morphodifferentiation	Bell stage	Proliferation of inner enamel epithelium to form shape of crown	Disorders of size and shape
Histodifferentiation		Differentiation of precursor cells into ameloblasts and odontoblasts	Regional odontodysplasia
Apposition	Crown stage	Reciprocal induction and laying down of mantle dentine and first enamel	Enamel hypoplasia
Calcification			Amelogenesis imperfecta Dentinogenesis imperfecta
Maturation		Enamel crystal growth	Enamel hypomineralisation
Eruption		Emergence of tooth and continued development of roots	Impacted teeth

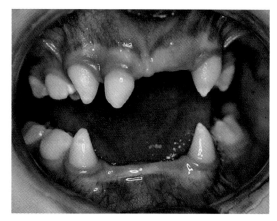

Figure 41.1 The typical appearance of a child with ectodermal dysplasia with multiple missing teeth and conical form of other teeth.

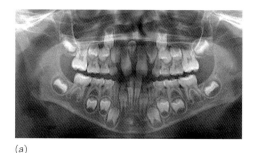

(a)

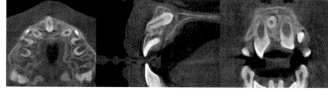

(b)

Figure 41.3 The advantages of using computerised tomography to aid in the localisation of a supernumerary tooth. (a) The panoramic film shows a midline tuberculate supernumerary. (b) Reconstruction films in axial, sagittal and coronal planes showing the relationship to the immature central incisors.

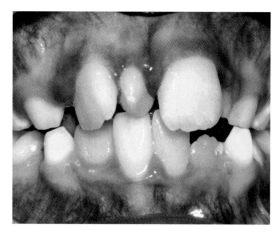

Figure 41.2 Conical supernumeraries usually erupt.

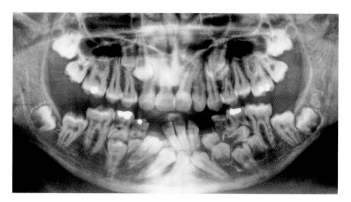

Figure 41.4 Radiographic appearance of cleidocranial dysplasia with multiple supernumerary teeth.

Paediatric Dentistry at a Glance, First Edition. Monty Duggal, Angus Cameron and Jack Toumba. © 2013 John Wiley & Sons Ltd. Published 2013 by Blackwell Publishing Ltd.

Hypodontia

There are many alternative terminologies for missing teeth, including hypodontia, oligodontia (only a few teeth) and anodontia (complete absence of teeth); and the absence of teeth is the most common dental anomaly with up to 9% of people affected. While the number of missing teeth is important, of more relevance is what type of tooth is absent. Table 41.1 shows the anomalies that exist at different stages of tooth development.

Commonly, the lateral incisors, second premolars or third molars are absent. It is rare to have absence of the first molars, canines or central incisors and further investigation is required to exclude possible syndromes or other congenital abnormalities.

Ectodermal dysplasias (ED) (Fig. 41.1)

This represents a group of conditions where any or all of the ectodermally derived tissues may be affected, including skin, nails, hair and teeth. The classical sex-linked hypohidrotic form affects boys most severely, with many missing teeth, fine sparse hair and the absence of sweat glands. Female carriers are less severely affected and are often diagnosed due to their hypodontia.

Management problems with hypodontia

- Aesthetics.
- Association with other dental anomalies (conical teeth).
- Diminished vertical dimension or lack of bilateral support.
- Speech and articulation disorders.
- Lack of adequate anchorage for conventional orthodontics.
- Impacted teeth due to lack of guidance for erupting teeth.

Treatment planning

Ultimately, every child is different and there must be an individualised plan for each patient, based on their social, functional and aesthetic needs. While some adolescents may be too young for complex treatment, the absence of teeth in this social age group is important and compromises and flexibility in treatment planning are needed.

- Early, long-term, multidisciplinary treatment planning.
- Growth and development and social implications.
- Definitive advanced restorative treatment when growth finished.
- Provide adequate aesthetics, bilateral support and function.

Management options

- Composite resin strip crowns or build-ups.
- Partial dentures.
- Orthodontic treatment to close spaces.
- Surgery may be required to manage impacted or ectopic teeth.
- Advanced restorative options including crowns, bridges and osseo-integrated implants once growth has finished.

Reshaping of teeth is an excellent option for conical teeth. Use composite resin in the growing child first rather than cast restorations. Orthodontic treatment planning should be undertaken early to consider the options as to when later treatment might commence. Children tolerate dentures extremely well, although denture design will differ (Adam's cribs for retention). Cobalt chromium denture frameworks are useful to decrease the thickness in the palate that will interfere with speech. In some children with ED, the provision of dentures might occur as early as 3–4 years of age.

Use of osseo-integrated implants in children

There is good evidence that modern implant technology is well suited to the management of children with missing teeth. Implants are well tolerated and undergo integration, but will behave like a submerging anklylosed tooth in a growing child. Implants are now being placed early in some children, in particular, those with anodontia and in the lower canine region.

Supernumerary teeth

These extra teeth arise from a budding of the dental lamina and affect up to 4% of the population. While a number of syndromes present with supernumerary teeth (cleidocranial dysplasia and Gardner's syndrome), most are sporadic (with an hereditary component) and 98% occur in the maxilla. Supernumeraries may be conical (Fig. 41.2) or tubercular in form.

Conical teeth usually erupt unless they are inverted and are commonly found in the midline of the maxilla (mesiodens). Tubercular forms are usually detected due to their blocking of the normal central incisor.

Localisation of supernumerary teeth

- Periapical and anterior maxillary occlusal films.
- Use of tube-shift techniques.
- 3D and cone-beam tomography (Fig. 41.3).

Management

- Erupted (usually conical) teeth only require simple extraction.
- Tuberculate impacted teeth usually require surgical removal.

Timing of removal

As a general rule, supernumerary teeth should be removed as early as possible, so that there is no interference to the eruption of the permanent teeth. As most extra teeth are only diagnosed when there is delayed eruption of a central incisor, invariably this tooth has been displaced, so surgery is usually indicated immediately. If a supernumerary is diagnosed by chance on a routine radiograph, the decision to remove must take into account the developmental age of the permanent teeth and any possible damage that surgery might cause. Preferably, crown formation should be complete prior to surgery.

Surgery

The surgical removal of most palatal supernumerary teeth requires an approach via a palatal flap. Localisation is essential to avoid any possible damage to the permanent tooth. If diagnosis is late, and the central incisor is severely displaced then surgical exposure of the incisor might accompany surgical removal of the supernumerary. Depending on its position, the bonding of orthodontic brackets or chains and traction are often needed to bring the incisor into alignment.

Cleidocranial dysplasia (Fig. 41.4)

This is a rare autosomal dominant condition usually presenting with multiple supernumerary teeth and a number of other anomalies such as hypoplasia or absence of the clavicles, frontal bossing, hypertelorism, midface deficiency and short stature.

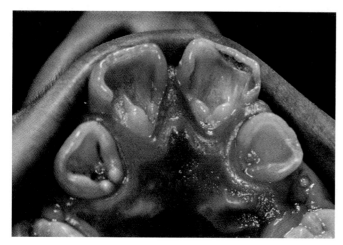

Figure 42.1 *Generalised macrodontia is uncommon. There is usually an accentuation of all the features of the crown particularly the marginal ridges giving the incisors a "shovel-shaped" appearance.*

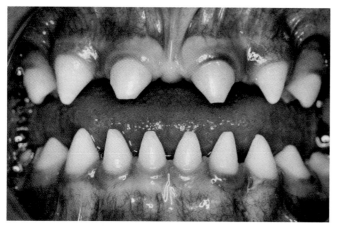

Figure 42.2 *Microdontia and conical teeth characteristically associated with ectodermal dysplasia.*

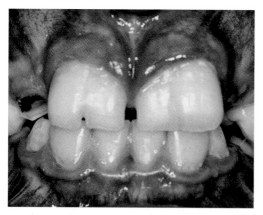

Figure 42.3 *The diagnosis of root canal morphology is important in the management of double teeth. This is a case of gemination with both the central incisors each having one large canal making surgical separation impossible.*

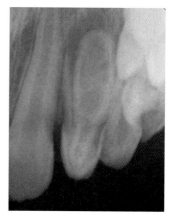

Figure 42.4 *A radiograph of the root canal morphology of a dens invaginatus. The prognosis of any treatment will depend on the ability to fully instrument and obturate this canal.*

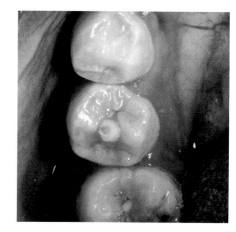

Figure 42.5 *A dens evaginatus in the lower second premolar of an Asian child. In this case the tubercle is still present and needs to be covered and protected to ensure that the pulp does not become necrotic.*

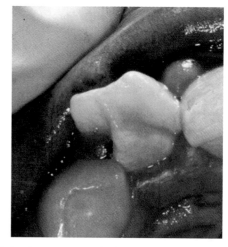

Figure 42.6 *A talon cusp commonly observed on the palatal surface of upper incisors.*

Paediatric Dentistry at a Glance, First Edition. Monty Duggal, Angus Cameron and Jack Toumba. © 2013 John Wiley & Sons Ltd. Published 2013 by Blackwell Publishing Ltd.

Changes in size and shape

Morphological anomalies occur during the morphodifferentiation stage of tooth development. Proliferation of the cells of the inner enamel epithelium results in changes in form of the teeth. While some anomalies have an hereditary component, most occur sporadically and the cause is unknown.

Macrodontia and microdontia

Macrodontia (Fig. 42.1)

Isolated macrodontia is associated with double teeth (see below) but generalised macrodontia is extremely rare. It may be associated with hormonal abnormalities such as pituitary giantism or developmental anomalies including hemifacial hyperplasia or KGB syndrome.

Management

Interproximal stripping may be possible depending on the size and position of the pulp chamber, but if the tooth is too large then extraction may be the only alternative followed by orthodontics and/or prosthodontic replacment.

Microdontia

Microdontia is commonly associated with cases of hypodontia, particularly with ectodermal dysplasia (Fig. 42.2). It is rare in the primary dentition and, while smaller teeth are more commonly found in females, macrodontia occurs more frequently in males. As with missing teeth, the last tooth in each series tends to be smaller in size. Generalised microdontia is extremely rare.

Management

• Composite resin veneers or build-ups.
• Orthodontic alignment.

Peg laterals

These are more commonly found in females, and are often associated with absence of the contralateral tooth. The smaller size of these teeth may result in failure of guidance for the canine resulting in palatal impaction. These teeth may be restored simply with a composite resin strip crown.

Double tooth (Fig. 42.3)

A relatively common anomaly in the primary dentition, this is a general term describing primary or permanent teeth that are joined together. Mostly incisors are affected.

Concrescence

This is fusion of two or more teeth by cementum.

Fusion

Fusion is joining of two teeth by dentine not involving pulp with two separate pulp canals. Tooth number may be reduced or normal if a supernumerary is fused to a normal tooth.

Gemination

Only one root canal is present. This usually represents twinning of a single tooth. In the permanent dentition these teeth are usually mac-

rodonts. Diagnosis of the root canal morphology may be aided by use of cone beam CT as plain films are difficult to interpret.

Management

In the primary dentition, the central groove often becomes carious as it is difficult to clean. Fused teeth are possible to surgically separate if separate root canals are present. These may then be moved orthodontically and reshaped to resemble normal teeth.

Geminated teeth are often impossible to reshape or reduce the size due to the position and large size of the root canal, and extraction is usually the only option. It is essential to involve an orthodontic assessment in treatment planning and, while some children may be ideally too young to commence complex treatment, the social impacts must be considered.

Dens invaginatus (Fig. 42.4)

Sometimes termed dens-in-dente, this anomaly is usually found in maxillary lateral incisors (but central incisors or premolars may also be affected) that have an exaggerated invagination of the cingulum pit. Following eruption, these teeth often become necrotic and the child may present with a canine fossa cellulitis. The ability to treat these teeth is dependent on the ability to not only instrument an extremely complex root canal, but ultimately obturate the canal. Extraction is commonly needed.

Dens evaginatus (Fig. 42.5)

This affects lower premolars often in Asian populations and is more common in females. A tubercle is present on the occlusal surface. The tooth often becomes exposed soon after eruption with fracture or abrasion of the tubercle exposing the pulp horn.

Management

• Protect the tubercle with composite resin or fissure sealing.
• Elective Cvek pulpotomy and removal of tubercle.
• If exposed, root canal therapy should be commenced and if the apex is immature, these are excellent cases for revascularisation techniques.

Talon cusp (Fig. 42.6)

The T-cingulum or talon cusp is an exaggerated cingulum of maxillary, usually permanent, incisors.

Management

• Often no treatment is required with no occlusal interference.
• Selective grinding of the cusp if interfering with occlusion.

Taurodontism

In this anomaly, there is an increased size of the pulp chamber, usually with a conical root and occurs frequently in a number of syndromes including:
• ectodermal dysplasias;
• X-linked vitamin D-resistant rickets;
• regional odontodysplasia;
• Klinefelter's syndrome.
No treatment is usually required.

Table 43.1 Discolouration of teeth.

Green	Localised extrinsic	Chromogenic bacteria
Black/grey	Localised extrinsic	Ferrous sulphate
	Localised intrinsic	Amalgam
	Generalised intrinsic	Necrotic pulp
White	Localised intrinsic	Developmental defect (trauma)
	Generalised intrinsic	Fluorosis
Brown	Localised extrinsic	Arrested caries or food stains
Yellow	Generalised extrinsic	Bile pigments from jaundice
Yellow brown	Generalised intrinsic	Amelogenesis imperfecta
Green/blue	Generalised intrinsic	Hyperbilirubinaemia
Blue/brown	Generalised intrinsic	Dentinogenesis imperfecta
Pink	Localised intrinsic	Internal resorption
Red/brown	Generalised Intrinsic	Porphyria

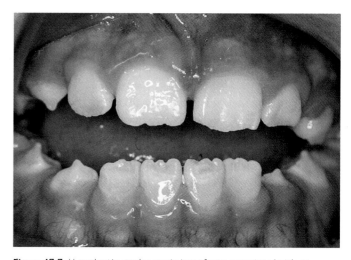

Figure 43.3 Hypoplastic amelogenesis imperfecta associated with an anterior open bite. This smooth form has very thin enamel that is of relatively normal quality. Note the spacing between the teeth and the accentuated cusp tips, especially on the canines.

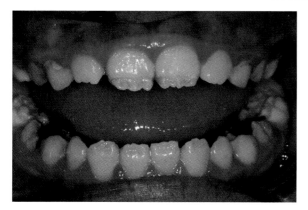

Figure 43.1 Chronological hypoplasia associated with a febrile illness in the first 12 months of life. This has led to damage to the ameloblasts secreting enamel at this time, affecting the teeth at different levels depending on their developmental stage.

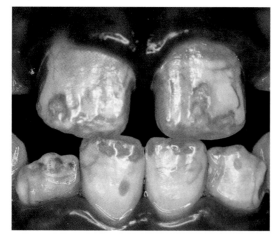

Figure 43.2 Mild to moderate fluorosis. This is a surface hypomineralisation limited to the outer 100 µm layer of the enamel. As such, this is a defect during the maturation stage of tooth development and may be treated with microabrasion. The primary teeth are unaffected.

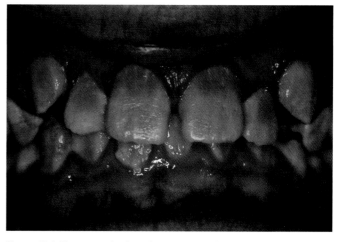

Figure 43.4 Hypomineralised amelogenesis imperfecta. The enamel is extremely soft and discoloured and there tends to be a build-up of calculus around the cervical region of the teeth.

Paediatric Dentistry at a Glance, First Edition. Monty Duggal, Angus Cameron and Jack Toumba. © 2013 John Wiley & Sons Ltd. Published 2013 by Blackwell Publishing Ltd.

Chronological disturbances

Teeth represent a fossil record of *in utero*, perinatal and childhood illness. Developmental defects of enamel can be acquired or inherited, localised to single teeth, generalised affecting the entire dentition or chronological affecting all teeth in different patterns dependent on the stage of formation of those teeth at the time of the insult. Tooth development begins at 3–4 months *in utero* and continues until the root formation of the third molars is complete. Any severe systemic upset may affect ameloblast function resulting in death of these cells, abnormalities in the secretion of enamel proteins, interrupted calcification or maturation of the enamel. This will result in the characteristic patterns of chronological hypoplasia affecting teeth at different stages of development (Fig. 43.1). *In utero* disturbances will cause defects in the primary dentition but the permanent teeth should be unaffected. Perinatal illness will affect the first permanent molars but the incisors should be unaffected as they do not begin to calcify until 3–4 months after birth.

Hypoplasia

Hypoplasia is a disorder in the quantity of the enamel. Hypoplastic enamel may also be hypomineralised but there are some teeth that are purely hypoplastic with no change in the quality of the enamel. This occurs during the secretory phase (apposition and calcification stages) of tooth development. Generally, composite resin will bond well to enamel that is deficient in quantity but poorly to hypomineralised enamel. Breakdown may occur very rapidly following tooth eruption and treatment of these teeth should not be delayed.

Hypomineralisation (opacities)

Hypomineralisation is a defect in the quality of the enamel. It occurs principally during the maturation phase of tooth development and results in incomplete enamel crystal growth or a cessation in prism formation. There may be an incorporation of pigments leading to discolouration (Table 43.1) or it may be simply an opacity that indicates air voids within the prism. Hypomineralised posterior teeth are extremely susceptible to caries and are often extremely sensitive.

Fluorosis

The presentation of fluorosis may range from very mild white flecking through the enamel (Fig. 43.2) to severe staining (mottling) and hypoplasia, depending on the dosage and exposure to fluoride. Approximately 10% of the population will manifest some visible forms of fluorosis at water concentrations of 1 ppm. This is usually limited to flecking or opacity through the enamel. It is extremely uncommon to observe fluorosis in the primary dentition.

Molar incisor hypomineralisation

This is a term used to describe a form of chronological hypoplasia/hypomineralisation affecting the first permanent molars with/or without defects on the permanent incisors. While some molars may be so malformed as to require extraction, teeth that are theoretically forming at the same time may be unaffected. Often there is no aetiological factor, however, it is important to go through a thorough pregnancy and perinatal history to exclude other causes.

Amelogenesis imperfecta (AI)

Amelogenesis imperfecta describes a range of inherited enamel deficiencies affecting both dentitions. At least four different mutations have been identified (several others probably exist) and transmission may be autosomal dominant, autosomal recessive or sex-linked, also exhibiting Lyonisation in hemizygous females. Despite the numerous classifications of AI, the enamel defects are predominately:

Hypoplastic (Fig. 43.3)
There is generalised thin enamel, which may be rough, smooth or pitted with spacing between teeth. Only pitted forms are prone to caries. It may also be associated with an anterior open bite and teeth may fail to erupt or undergo resorption.

Hypomineralised (Fig. 43.4)
The enamel is initially normal in form but softer. It is discoloured (yellow/brown), often prone to caries and in severe forms enamel may be so soft that it can be scraped away.

Management of enamel defects

In general, the aims of management are to treat pathology and pain, provide adequate aesthetic appeal, maintain occlusal function and maintain the vertical dimension. One of the major difficulties with newly erupted hypoplastic teeth is that they may be exquisitely sensitive.

- Glass ionomer cement as an interim restoration.
- Full coverage with stainless steel crowns.
- Extraction of hopeless teeth early (timed with an orthodontic opinion).
- Small superficial opacities may be treated with microabrasion using a multifluted tungsten carbide bur, an acid abrasion technique. Deep stains extending through the enamel may require removal of the stain and replacement with composite resin.
- Composite resin will bond normally to purely hypoplastic enamel but poorly to hypomineralised enamel. Use resin veneers, strip crowns and crown build-ups or indirect resin crowns.
- Stainless steel crowns are invaluable in the management of cases of AI or teeth with generalised hypoplasia. Consider placing crowns early to limit attrition and maintain the vertical dimension of the occlusion. This may also preserve and limit wear to the anterior teeth.
- Delay definitive advanced restorative work, with porcelains for example, until growth has ceased, but always consider and do not compromise on the social needs of the child particularly through adolescence. The best clinical results on posterior permanent teeth come with the use of cast metal onlays or stainless steel crowns.

Other considerations
- Genetic counselling to determine a correct diagnosis.
- Early orthodontic assessment and multidisciplinary planning.
- Children with inherited disorders require a lifetime of dental treatment and it is important to consider the long-term prognosis of work and keep options open.

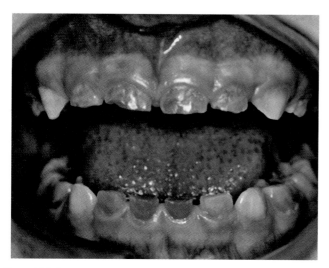

Figure 44.1 Dentinogenesis imperfecta with the typical appearance of grey–bluish opalescence of the teeth with enamel present and yellow–brown exposed dentine.

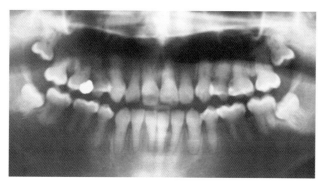

Figure 44.2 Classical appearance of an adolescent with dentinogenesis imperfecta. Note the bulbous crowns and shortened roots. Over time the initially wide-open apices and thin root canals become obliterated.

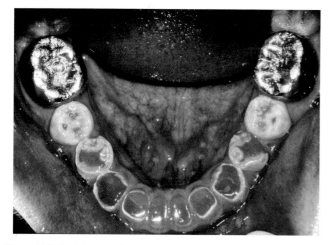

Figure 44.3 Stainless steel crowns are invaluable in the restoration of these teeth. Once the enamel is lost the dentine wears rapidly making long-term retention poor.

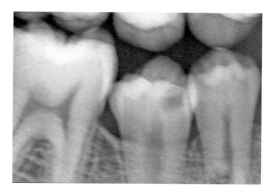

Figure 44.4 A pre-eruptive intracoronal defect of dentine in a lower second premolar. There is no caries and the enamel surface is intact.

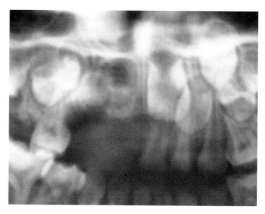

Figure 44.5 A case of regional odontodysplasia affecting the upper right incisors. Note the difference in appearance of the contralateral teeth. This gives rise to the term "ghost teeth".

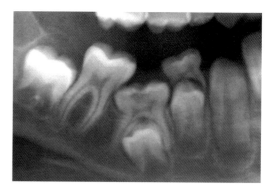

Figure 44.6 Ankylosis of the lower second primary molar. Sometimes it may be the case that these teeth have never erupted. The first permanent molar has erupted over the, now carious, primary tooth. The lack of proximal contact has resulted in space loss making removal difficult. It is preferable to distalise the permanent molar prior to surgically removing the primary tooth. A space maintainer is then needed to allow adequate space into which the second premolar can erupt.

Paediatric Dentistry at a Glance, First Edition. Monty Duggal, Angus Cameron and Jack Toumba. © 2013 John Wiley & Sons Ltd. Published 2013 by Blackwell Publishing Ltd.

Inherited disorders of dentine

All the different anomalies of dentine are inherited and are principally related to disorders of collagen metabolism but are phenotypically very similar.

Dentinogenesis imperfecta (DI) and hereditary opalescent dentine

These are inherited disorders of dentine and collagen metabolism. Clinically identical conditions, the term dentinogenesis imperfecta is usually reserved for the condition associated with osteogenesis imperfecta and hereditary opalescent dentine for the isolated condition. The appearance is characteristic with an amber or grey to blue opalescent colour of the crown (Fig. 44.1). The enamel is normal but will chip and expose the weaker and abnormal dentine that wears rapidly. Over time there is pulp canal obliteration and radiographically the crowns are bulbous (Fig. 44.2).

Management

It is essential that the enamel of these teeth is protected and early placement of stainless steel crowns on primary molars is recommended (Fig. 44.3). The anterior teeth may be built up with composite resin strip crowns although over time these are lost and some form of full-coverage restoration is required. Initially, the appearance of the permanent dentition is good, however, these teeth tend to deteriorate in early adult life necessitating complex restorative work throughout a lifetime.

Osteogenesis imperfecta (OI)

OI is an uncommon inherited connective tissue disease of type I collagen characterised by severe bone fragility, blue sclera and dentinogenesis imperfecta. Four different types have been described all with variable expression of the mutation. In severe forms, the children suffer from multiple long-bone fractures and are often confined to wheelchairs. Fractures of the facial bones are extremely uncommon.

Dentinal dysplasia (DD)

Two different forms of dentinal dysplasia are now recognised:
- coronal dentinal dysplasia;
- radicular dentinal dysplasia.

Both are inherited conditions but there is general agreement that coronal DD is a form of dentinogenesis imperfecta. In the long term, children with radicular DD will usually lose their teeth due to a lack of support and spontaneous abscess formation. The management of coronal DD is similar to that of dentinogenesis imperfecta.

Vitamin D-resistant rickets

This is an uncommon sex-linked condition also termed hypophosphataemic rickets that causes changes in the long bones due to a failure of renal distal tubular reabsorption of phosphate. Affected children have features similar to classical rickets with short stature and bowed legs but there are also dentinal changes with abnormalities of the pulp chamber and multiple spontaneous abscesses in the primary dentition.

These children require pre-emptive treatment with placement of prophylactic stainless steel crowns to prevent enamel wear and exposure of any dentine that will lead to pulp necrosis.

Pre-eruptive intracoronal resorptive defects

These are often found on routine radiographic surveys as an isolated radiolucency in the dentine independent of any abnormality in the enamel (Fig. 44.4). While these lesions do not appear to expand over time, it is recommended that they be treated once the tooth has erupted by opening into the lesion and restoration with glass ionomer cement and composite resin.

Regional odontodysplasia

Often described as "ghost teeth" (Fig. 44.5), this rare condition is sporadic and characterised by abnormal development of both enamel and dentine that is localised to one or several teeth in one area of an arch. The enamel and dentine are grossly hypoplastic and once erupted these teeth usually become necrotic and abscessed. The aetiology is unknown although a microvascular defect has been proposed. While these teeth may be managed initially with stainless crowns, invariably these teeth require extraction.

Disorders of eruption

There is very little correlation between somatic development and the emergence of the teeth. The average age for the appearance of the first tooth is 6–7 months, however, some children may be born with teeth while others may not have any teeth erupted until after 12 months of age. What is more important than the timing of eruption is the sequence of eruption and a consistent developmental progression. Precocious eruption of the permanent dentition is very uncommon and if associated with the early exfoliation of the primary teeth, then these children should be investigated for probability of systemic pathology (see Chapter 40).

Ankylosed primary molars (Fig. 44.6)

Commonly, primary molars are observed to submerge into the gingiva. There is controversy as to whether these teeth are truly ankylosed, nonetheless, it appears that there may also be a failure or cessation of resorption of the primary tooth. Essentially, the primary tooth retains its position while the surrounding teeth will move with the growth of the alveolus giving the appearance of submergence. Most teeth will migrate mesially over time and, with the eruption of the first permanent molar, there is a concomitant loss of space and the primary molar becomes impacted. It is important to try to regain and retain space initially.

The decision to extract or surgically remove the primary molar will depend on:
- the depth of the primary tooth in the alveolus;
- the presence of any caries in this tooth;
- whether there is any normal physiological root resorption;
- the position and development of the permanent tooth;
- the amount of space in the arch or other orthodontic considerations.

Box 45.1 Conditions/diseases associated with learning disability (Scully and Cawson, 2005)

Chromosomal anomalies
- Fragile X syndrome
- Autosomal trisomies (Edwards' syndrome, Patau's syndrome, Down syndrome)
- Deletions 5, short arm (cri du chat syndrome)
- Deletions 4, short arm (Wolf's syndrome)
- Sex chromosome anomalies (XO Turner's syndrome, XXX superfemale, XXY Klinefelter's syndrome, XYY syndromes)

Inborn errors of metabolism
- Protein:
  - Hypothyroidism (cretinism)
  - Phenylketonuria
  - Homocystinuria
  - Wilson's disease
- Carbohydrate:
  - Galactosaemia
  - Mucopolysaccharidosis
- Lipids:
  - Tay–Sachs disease
  - Gaucher's disease
- Purines:
  - Lesch–Nyhan syndrome

Phakomatoses (neurocutaneous disorders)
- Neurofibromatosis (von Recklinghausen's disease)
- Encephalofacial angiomatosis (Sturge–Weber syndrome)
- Tuberous sclerosis (epilopia)

Microcephaly

Intrauterine damage (e.g. hypoxia)

Prematurity

Intrauterine infections
- Cytomegalovirus
- HIV
- Rubella
- Syphilis
- Toxoplasmosis

Radiation

Acquired causes of learning disability
- Trauma
- Hypoxia
- Alzheimer's disease
- Meningitis, encephalitis, HIV
- Metabolic disorders
- Poisons
- Rhesus incompatibility

Paediatric Dentistry at a Glance, First Edition. Monty Duggal, Angus Cameron and Jack Toumba. © 2013 John Wiley & Sons Ltd. Published 2013 by Blackwell Publishing Ltd.

Definition

Learning disability has been described as "a significant impairment of intelligence and social functioning acquired before adulthood". An intelligence quotient of less than 70 has been used as the arbitrary dividing line that defines learning disability There are a number of medical conditions/diseases that are associated with learning disability and these are summarised in Box 45.1.

Provision of oral health care

Services provided for people with learning disabilities should aim to improve their quality of life and help them achieve their fullest potential in society. Dental services for these children should aim to reduce the number of dental symptoms, maintain oral function and therefore their perception of oral well-being and quality of life. Regardless of nature or extent of the disability, everyone has equal rights and therefore dental services should be provided in a way that:

* recognises that they are individuals;
* recognises their right to participate in decisions that affect their lives;
* provides the amount of support necessary to enable everyday living, including adequate health care.

Overcoming specific problems in oral care

Provision of routine oral care can be challenging for the carers due to:
* lack of cooperation;
* strong tongue thrust;
* gagging on brushing.

Various aids are available to overcome these problems, but a tailor-made approach is required for each individual child.

Some useful tips for effective brushing

* To distract the child, allow to bite on a toothbrush whilst the teeth are cleaned with another toothbrush.
* Finger shields that have a small head of soft latex tufts are available and may be useful.
* A flannel or gauze-square wrapped around the forefinger to gently retract or hold back the tongue or lip may be used in those with a strong tongue thrust.
* It may be helpful to start brushing from the back teeth and move forward in those with strong gag reflex.
* A different area of the mouth can be brushed on different occasions keeping note of the area brushed each time so several short brushing sessions can be used. Other distractions such as music and videos can be used.
* Holding hands or lying a small child back into the lap may be required, with help from another person.
* Above all patience and perseverance are needed and full involvement of the parents or carers of the child is important. They know the child the best and the child usually responds much better to the regular carer.

Specific oral complications

Drooling. This can result in chronic irritation of the facial skin, increase in peri-oral infections, halitosis and dehydration due to fluid loss. Assessment should be made by a multidisciplinary team. Non-surgical approaches to manage drooling could include maintaining an upright head position, bio-feedback techniques, bio-functional therapy, behavioural therapy and physiotherapy. Sometimes functional appliances to improve swallowing and chewing in people with cerebral palsy are used. Pharmacological treatments and rarely surgery can be considered.

Bruxism. This can lead to exposed dentine and may cause pain and infection. Provision of bite guards may be helpful but needs individual assessment.

Erosion. Acid reflux is a common problem and tooth surface loss is a combination of bruxism and reflux of acid in the mouth. Appropriate consultation with the patient's doctor or referral to a specialist is necessary. In many cases full coverage of primary and permanent molars with stainless steel crowns is required.

Dry mouth. Dry mouth can lead to decay, infection of the oral mucosa and periodontal disease. Management includes:
* saliva replacements;
* the use of sugar-free chewing gum and sugar-free fluids can be advised depending on severity of the disability;
* regular professional application of fluorides such as fluoride varnish.

Self-injurious behaviour. May be linked to cerebral palsy, or disorders such as Lesch–Nyhan syndrome or Riley Day syndrome. Construction of mouthguards or other oral appliances should be considered. Distraction and behavioural psychology is a useful management option. In some cases extractions are required to protect a child from self-harm.

People with feeding difficulties who are tube-fed. This group of people includes those fed by gastrostomy, jejunostomy and nasogastric tube. There is a lack of coordination of swallowing with breathing. An inadequately protected airway increases the risk of gastric reflux causing aspiration, which leads to recurrent bouts of pneumonia. Treatment under GA is frequently required.

Use of sedation and GA

Factors to be considered in the use of sedation or GA in this group of patients are age and medical condition, cultural acceptance of sedation, behaviour management problems, support from carers, experience and training of dental team in sedation techniques.

Pre-assessment. A full, updated medical history, including past anaesthetic history, should be obtained from the patient's doctor. Provide clear instructions of the planned procedure to the patient or carer in order to allay anxieties. Pre-medication should be considered. Ensure the correct consent form is completed. For those unable to give consent, this will require a case discussion involving the multidisciplinary team, the patient's key worker and next of kin.

Anatomical considerations. Many congenital and developmental disabilities are associated with facial and oral abnormalities. It is important that the airway of the patient is properly assessed by the anaesthetist. A poor dentition could pose an additional problem during induction. The anaesthetist should also be made aware of problems associated with cleft palate and enlarged tongue.

The anaesthetic. Discussions should take place between the anaesthetist and the dental team regarding the patient. Arrangements must be made with ward and day surgery unit staff to make sure they understand the needs of people with learning disabilities. If people with learning disabilities are sharing a ward with other patients, appointments need to be carefully arranged to minimise any disruption that might be experienced.

Social factors in assessment. Arrangements for effective and efficient after care should be in place.

Dental treatment under GA

For dental treatment under GA, a rational treatment plan should be made, which might be more radical than normal. Any teeth of doubtful prognosis should be extracted rather than restored with the risk that the patient would need another GA were the treatment to fail.

46 Physical and learning disabilities II

Box 46.1 Oral/dental features of Down syndrome

Soft tissue
- Open mouth posture due to the underdevelopment of the middle third of the face and poor muscle tone
- The tongue may be absolutely or relatively large and is often fissured, protrusive (tongue thrust)
- Lips tend to be thick, dry and fissured
- High incidence of severe, periodontal disease
- Palate often appears to be high, with horizontal palatal shelves but a short palate is more characteristic
- May exhibit congenital deformities such as bifid uvula, cleft lip and cleft palate

Hard tissue
- Anterior open bite, posterior crossbite and other types of malocclusion common
- Maxilla is small and mandible is somewhat relatively protrusive
- Delayed development and eruption of teeth
- Hypodontia, with upper laterals and third molars missing most commonly
- Microdontia (in 30–50% of the cases)
- Hypocalcification and hypoplastic defects
- Low caries activity usually
- Short, small crowns and roots of teeth
- Parafunctional habit

Functional disorders
- Difficulties in swallowing, speech and mastication

Box 46.2 Subclassification of cerebral palsy according to nature of motor disorder

I. **Spastic CP:** 70–80% of cases. Its predominant characteristic is increased muscle tone

Quadriplegia: all four extremities, the trunk, and oromotor musculature are involved

Diplegia: spasticity in the legs. Arms also can be affected but to a lesser extent. Approximately 50% of these cases are associated with preterm birth

Hemiplegia: one side of the body is involved

Monoplegia: extremely rare, only one limb is involved

II. **Dyskinetic CP:** 10–15% of cases. Motor characteristics include hypotonia, overall problems with coordination, oromotor difficulties, including speech and swallowing difficulties

III. **Ataxic CP:** 5% of cases. These individuals have problems with voluntary movement, balance and depth perception

Box 46.3 Barriers to access and provision of oral care

Access
- Lack of perceived need
- Inability to express need
- Lack of ability for self-care
- Inadequate training of support workers in oral health
- Lack of training and experience of clinicians

Communication
- Restricted ability to communicate
- Lack the verbal skills
- Inability to convey fear and anxiety
- Withdrawal, and aggression towards self and others
- Clinician's dependence on carers for communication

Consent and capacity
- The consenting parent must fully understand the procedure
- Where carer unable to consent, it is possible for a court to give that consent
- The ability and understanding of the proposed treatment by the child has to be taken into consideration before proceeding with the treatment, particularly in older children
- It is important to assess capacity and follow national laws

Paediatric Dentistry at a Glance, First Edition. Monty Duggal, Angus Cameron and Jack Toumba. © 2013 John Wiley & Sons Ltd. Published 2013 by Blackwell Publishing Ltd.

Down syndrome

Down syndrome (DS), the most common cause of mild–moderate learning disability, is a chromosomal anomaly that results from the presence of an additional third chromosome 21. Due to its characteristic appearance and chromosomal disorder, Down syndrome has also been known as mongolism or trisomy 21. The incidence varies between one in 800 to 1000 live births. Increasing life expectancy of affected individuals means that most dentists will be called upon to treat children and adults with DS.

Learning disability is a universal feature of DS although the degree of learning disability in DS patients differs from individual to individual. However, most are able to communicate well and live semi-independently.

The oral/dental features are shown in Box 46.1.

Specific management issues
Behaviour management

Most DS children are amicable and can be managed with local analgesia with or without inhalation sedation, and good behaviour management. However, for the uncooperative DS patient, treatment under general anaesthesia may have to be considered. General anaesthesia, if required, should be administered by a specialist in a hospital. There is increased risk involved for DS patients due to the cardiac defects, intubation difficulties, increased susceptibility to respiratory infections and possibility of atlanto-axial subluxation.

Cardiac problems

Congenital heart defects (CHDs) affect around 40% of DS infants. The child may suffer from early pulmonary hypertension if the defect is large. Careful liaison with the paediatrician is essential. For patients who have no history of cardiac examination, it would be prudent to have one arranged before providing invasive dental treatment. If a CHD is found follow protocols described in Chapter 49.

Periodontal disease

DS patients have increased prevalence of periodontal disease, due to compromised immunity and poor oral hygiene.

Malocclusion

Crossbites, anterior open bites and class III malocclusion are often present. Microdontia and hypodontia are occasional features.

Dental caries

Caries assessment should be routinely performed. There is some evidence that the prevalence of dental caries is low due to a higher salivary pH, low *Streptococcus mutans* counts, microdontia, hypodontia, spaced dentition and shallow fissures in premolars and molars.

Dental management

A realistic preventive programme that encompasses all the important features of preventive dentistry should be developed with particular emphasis on management of the periodontal health.

Autistic spectrum disorder (ASD)

Autism is a lifelong developmental disability that becomes evident in infancy, usually within the first 3 years of life. It affects the areas of the brain that control language, social interaction and creative and abstract thinking, and affects the way a person communicates with, and relates to, people and the world around them. Autism affects about 1 or 2 people in every 100 in the UK and is more common in boys than girls with a ratio of 3.5:1.

Dental management

- The National Autistic Society (NAS) advises carers to compile "a social story book" of photos or pictures for use at home, to show the stages of visiting the dentist from the moment the patient leaves home for the dentist, as this may help the patient know what to expect next. The NAS recommends including a "reward picture" at the end (such as a favourite activity) so the patient knows there is something to look forward to. Generally, it is better to inform the child of the visit as early as possible.
- Use clear, simple language with short sentences and use direct requests.
- Develop a routine in which the child is not kept waiting and has a short quiet visit, including being seen by the same dental staff. Patients with autism may be disturbed by the noise in the dental office such as air rotor or aspirator, so treatment under local anaesthesia may be impossible. General anaesthesia is often required.

Cerebral palsy

Cerebral palsy (CP) is the most common congenital neuromuscular handicap resulting from damage to the brain early in the course of its development: during foetal development, during the birth process or during the first few months after birth. The motor disorders of cerebral palsy are often accompanied by disturbances of sensation, cognition, communication, perception, behaviour and/or a seizure disorder. Prevalence is 2–3 per 1000 live births. Types of CP are described in Box 46.2.

Dental management

The specific issues related to children with CP are related to access, communication/behaviour, involuntary movements, and also the seizure disorders. It is possible to provide simple routine care for many children with CP without GA with the help of the carers, who can be very helpful in the management of the child. However, GA or IV sedation administered by an anaesthetist is very often required to provide comprehensive care, including periodontal care. Specific concerns regarding use of GA/sedation can be:
- scoliosis can affect a patient's ventilatory capacity;
- a compromised gag reflex can put a patient at more risk for aspiration;
- joint contractures may make patient positioning difficult;
- poorly controlled seizures can complicate sedation.

Barriers to access and provision of oral care in children with physical and learning disabilities are summarised in Box 46.3.

Table 47.1 Special investigations for children with suspected bleeding disorders.

Full blood count	Will identify thrombocytopenia and anaemia which could have been induced through haemorrhage
Clotting screen	Required in all cases
Prothrombin time	Measures effectiveness of extrinsic pathway factors I, II, V, VII, IX, X Increased in warfarin or heparin therapy
INR	Patient's thrombin time divided by normal thrombin time (normal=1) Required for all children on warfarin who require invasive dental treatment
Activated partial thromboplastin time (APTT)	Is increased in the haemophilias, von Willebrand's disease and deficiency of factors XI and XII
Thrombin time	Increased in parenchymal liver disease
Group and save	If possibility of prolonged haemorrhage is anticipated blood sample can be grouped facilitating requests for blood or blood products at short notice
Cross match	If severe haemorrhage is expected a number of units can be cross matched

Table 47.2 Dental management of children with haemophilia A.

Dental care/precautions	Drugs that may be required
Regular check up and rigorous prevention	Factor VIII cover is required for dental extractions and surgery, as well as for inferior
Buccal infiltrations with 4% articaine, 1:100 000 epinephrine, may be given instead of inferior alveolar nerve block	alveolar nerve blocks and lingual infiltrations
Soft tissue manipulation and trauma kept to a minimum	In all but severe haemophiliacs most other dental treatment can be performed using antifibrinolytic agents such as tranexamic acid. These can be used systemically as
Rubber dam clamp placed as atraumatically as possible	tablets but also as mouthwash for topical effect
High volume aspiration used carefully as may cause haematoma	Desmopressin (DDAVP) given as an intravenous infusion, subcutaneous injection or

Orthodontic treatment should avoid sharp edges to minimise soft
   tissue trauma
	intranasally, induces release of factor VIIIC, vWF and tissue plasminogen activator
	   (tPA), and may also be used to aid haemostasis

	Always communicate with haematologist

Paediatric Dentistry at a Glance, First Edition. Monty Duggal, Angus Cameron and Jack Toumba. © 2013 John Wiley & Sons Ltd. Published 2013 by Blackwell Publishing Ltd.

Introduction

Patients with bleeding disorders are at an increased risk from certain dental procedures. The principles of safe dental management of these patients are:
- accurate diagnosis from appropriate history, examination and special tests (Table 47.1);
- intensive prevention and regular review;
- careful preoperative planning and communication;
- use of appropriate local measures;
- careful prescribing;
- appropriate post-operative care.

Inherited coagulation defects

Haemophilia A

Haemophilia A is an X-linked recessive deficiency in factor VIII, whose prevalence is around 1 in 20000. The degree of severity is varied:
- severe (<1 IU/dl of factor VIII – normal range 50–100 IU/dl);
- moderate to severe (2–5 IU/dl);
- mild (6–40 IU/dl);
- carriers are treated as mild haemophiliacs if factor VIII levels are <50 IU/dl;
- factor VIII inhibitors. Around 20% of haemophiliacs who have had multiple transfusions develop inhibitory antibodies, which reduce the activity of factor VIII. Those with high titres of inhibitors require even greater care, such as immune-suppressant therapy or recombinant factor VIII.

Principles of dental management

Detailed management is shown in Table 47.2. As a general rule:
- **Severe and moderate haemophilia.** Treatment carried out in hospital environment, or with special arrangements having been made with the haemophilia unit in Community General Dental Practice.
- **Mild haemophilia.** Do not require all treatment to be carried out in hospital, but require close liaison with haemophilia unit.

Haemophilia B (Christmas disease)

Haemophilia B is a congenital factor IX deficiency, is less common than haemophilia A (1 in 50000 males) and is also inherited by the X-linked recessive manner. Female carriers often have a bleeding tendency.

Principles of dental management

- Patients require pre-operative factor IX replacement.
- Desmopressin is not used.
- Management is otherwise similar to that of haemophilia A.

Inherited disorders of platelet function

Von Willebrand's disease

This is the most common inherited bleeding disorder (1 : 1000). There is a deficiency of, or defect in, von Willebrand factor (vWF). This factor normally acts as a carrier for factor VIII, protecting it from proteolytic degradation. There is defective platelet function and coagulation.

Principles of dental management

- Liaise with haematologist.
- In most cases desmopressin (DDAVP) and/or an antifibrinolytic agent such as tranexamic acid is sufficient.
- However, in some rare variants such as types IIB and III, DDAVP is contra-indicated and factor VIII replacement is required. Antifibrinolytics, cryoprecipitate or fresh frozen plasma may also be required as well as local measures. Check with haematologist.

Thrombocytopenia

Thrombocytopenia is generally said to exist when the platelet count falls below 100×10^9/l, when petechiae, ecchymoses and post-operative haemorrhage may be present. A platelet count of less than 25×10^9/l is life threatening, and minor surgery should not be attempted if the platelet count is less than 50×10^9/l.

Principles of dental management

- In patients with idiopathic thrombocytopenic purpura (ITP), pre-operative treatment with oral prednisolone (4 mg/kg per day for 7 days) usually results in sufficient levels of platelets.
- In some forms of thrombocytopenia or disorders of platelet function, platelet transfusion may be required, but this should be avoided when possible, due to the risks of iso-immunisation, blood-borne viruses and rarely graft-versus-host disease.

Anticoagulated children

Most outpatients who are anticoagulated take warfarin, which is a vitamin K antagonist.

Principles of dental management

- Do not change the patient's warfarin therapy without discussion with the paediatrician.
- Minor oral surgery can be performed safely as long as the INR is <3.5 and appropriate local measures are used.
- Be aware of drug interactions of warfarin with drugs such as azole antifungals, metronidazole and non-steroidal anti-inflammatory drugs (NSAIDs) amongst others.

Some local measures

- Atraumatic technique.
- Epinephrine-containing LA.
- Sutures.
- Surgicel.
- Bone wax.
- Vacuum-formed splints.
- Coe-pak.
- Bipolar diathermy.

Post-operative care

- Don't discharge until haemostasis certain.
- Consider post-operative antibiotics.
- Soft diet.
- Avoid hot drinks.
- Avoid exercise.
- Post-operative tranexamic acid required frequently.
- Avoid aspirin/NSAIDs.

48 Thalassaemia and other blood dyscrasias

Box 48.1 Classification of blood dyscrasias

I. **Red blood cell disorders**
   a. **Anaemia**
      i) iron deficiency
      ii) glucose 6-phosphate dehydrogenase deficiency
      iii) sickle cell
      iv) thalassaemia
   b. **Polycythaemia**

II. **White blood cell disorders**
   a. **Leucocytosis**
      i) infectious mononucleosis (glandular fever)
      ii) neoplasia
   b. **Leucopenia = neutropenia**
      i) congenital
      ii) drug-induced
   c. **Leukaemias**
      i) acute lymphocytic (ALL)
      ii) acute myeloid (AML)
      iii) chronic
   d. **Lymphomas**
      i) Hodgkin's
      ii) Non-Hodgkin's
      iii) Burkitt's

Table 48.1 Possible oral manifestations of sickle cell anaemia and thalassaemia.

Sickle cell anaemia	Thalassaemia
Clinical	**Clinical**
• Infarcts in jaws can cause pain which may be mistaken for toothache or osteomyelitis	• Enlargement of the maxilla caused by bone marrow expansion
• Delayed skeletal maturation and delayed eruption	• There might be increased overjet and spacing of the maxillary incisors
• Mucosal pallor	• Painful swelling of the parotids
• Enamel hypomineralisation	• Xerostomia caused by iron deposition
• Asymptomatic pulpal necrosis has been reported. Sickle cells can cause a blockage of the blood vessels supplying the pulp, which can result in necrosis	• Sore or burning tongue related to the folate deficiency
	• Increased risk of caries due to xerostomia
Radiological	**Radiological**
• Increased radiolucency of the jaws due to decreased number of trabeculae	• Expansion of the diploe of the skull causes a hair-on-end appearance on lateral skull radiographs
• Enlarged marrow spaces	• Chicken-wire appearance due to alveolar bone rarefaction
• Cephalometric analyses of these patients indicate a tendency for a protrusive maxilla, forward advancement of the mandible and retroclined maxillary and mandibular incisors	• The lamina dura may be thin and the roots may be short
• Generalised osteoporosis	

Paediatric Dentistry at a Glance, First Edition. Monty Duggal, Angus Cameron and Jack Toumba. © 2013 John Wiley & Sons Ltd. Published 2013 by Blackwell Publishing Ltd.

Introduction

Dentists will often treat children who suffer from blood dyscrasias (Box 48.1). It is essential to have a knowledge of the commonly encountered conditions, their oral manifestations and the precautions required for their dental management.

Anaemia

Anaemia is characterised by a reduction in the oxygen-carrying capacity of the blood. It is usually related to a decrease in the number of circulating red blood cells (RBCs) or to an abnormality in the Hb contained within the RBCs.

Anaemia is not a disease but rather a symptom that may result from:
- decreased production of RBCs (iron deficiency, pernicious anaemia, folate deficiency);
- blood loss or increased rate of destruction of circulating RBCs that may cause haemolytic anaemia.

Haemolytic anaemias may result from many other causes including:
- inherited abnormal haemoglobin (the haemoglobinopathies);
- inherited abnormal structure or function of the erythrocyte such as spherocytosis, G6PD deficiency;
- damage to erythrocytes.

Dental management

- Safely managed with local anaesthesia.
- Implications for treatment under GA for those with severe anaemia. Pre-operative correction of haemoglobin levels are recommended. Liaise with haematologist and anaesthetist.

Sickle cell disorders

- Autosomal recessive inheritance.
- Affects mainly people of African, Afro-Caribbean, Mediterranean and Asian descent.

The life span of red blood cells is reduced from an average 120 days to 20 days and in those with homozygous sickle cell disease they become sickle-shaped when blood experiences lowered oxygen tension, decreased pH or when the patient becomes dehydrated. The outcome is erythrostasis, increased blood viscosity, reduced blood flow, hypoxia, increased adhesion of RBCs, vascular occlusion leading gradually to sickling crisis.

Sickle cell trait. Heterozygous state of the abnormal haemoglobin S (HbAS) which is more common. Frequently asymptomatic, but sickle cell crises can be caused by low oxygen tension (e.g. general anaesthesia). Can be treated as normal patients, except when carrying out GA when anaesthetist should be aware. Treat infections rigorously.

Sickle cell anaemia. Homozygous state of the abnormal haemoglobin S (HbSS). This is a serious disease with widespread complications becoming apparent about the third month of life. It presents four main problems:
- crises;
- chronic anaemia;
- chronic hyperbilirubinaemia;
- predisposition to infections.

Dental management

- Prefer to treat under local anaesthesia with or without sedation. Inhalation sedation is safe if oxygen levels are kept over 50%.
- Short appointments to minimise stress reduces the risk of crisis.
- Restorations should be preferred to extractions.
- Rigorous preventive dental care.

- Aspirin is best avoided as it can cause acidosis. Paracetamol and codeine are preferred.
- If patient is immunocompromised due to non-functional spleen, antibiotics (ABs) should be given for major surgical procedures.
- Benzodiazepines and other sedatives agents should be avoided.

Special care for treatment under GA

GA should be carried out only in hospital with full anaesthetic facilities and blood available for transfusion. At least 30% O_2 is needed and provided that there is no respiratory depression or obstruction anaesthetic procedures can be used.

If a crisis develops O_2 is given and bicarbonate infused. A packed red cell transfusion may be needed if the haemoglobin falls below 50%. Elective surgery should be carried out in hospital when haemolysis is minimal. It is best if anaemia is corrected pre-operatively and the haemoglobin is brought up to at least 10 g/dl.

Exchange transfusion is occasionally required for major surgery but only in selected patients. Prophylactic antimicrobials such as penicillin V or clindamycin should be given for surgical procedures and infections must be treated vigorously.

Thalassaemias

- Autosomal recessive inheritance.
- Either the α or β globin chains are synthesised at low rates leading to reduced production of haemoglobin A. The unaffected chains are produced in excess and precipitate within the erythrocytes to cause excessive erythrocyte fragility and haemolysis.

Heterozygous beta-thalassaemia (thalassaemia minor or thalassaemia trait) is common and usually asymptomatic except for mild hypochromic anaemia.

Homozygous beta-thalassaemia (Cooley's anaemia or thalassaemia major) is the most severe type and is characterised by failure to thrive, severe anaemia, hepatosplenomegaly and skeletal abnormalities. Some oral manifestations that can be associated with sickle cell anaemia and thalassaemia major are shown in Table 48.1.

Dental management

- Local anaesthesia is safe (lignocaine 1:80000 epinephrine can be used).
- Inhalation sedation may be given, keeping the O_2 level at least 40%.
- GA may be complicated due to enlargement of the maxilla, which may cause difficulties in intubation. Chronic severe anaemia and often cardiomyopathy are contraindications.
- Full blood count (FBC) and haemoglobin electrophoresis are required for patients at risk, if GA is to be given.
- If patient has a splenectomy, long-term ABs must be given (in liaison with paediatrician) for surgical procedures.
- Effective preventive measures, as patients with thalassaemia major are at high risk of developing caries according to studies.

Cyclic neutropenia

There is a periodic decrease in the number of neutrophils (about every 21–28 days). During the time of a low neutrophil count, children can experience symptoms which include fever without an obvious cause, ulcers of the mouth, sore throat, enlarged lymph nodes, skin infections, and even more serious infections due to this important part of the immune system being limited. Children with cyclic neutropenia suffer from periodontal disease characterised by generalised bone loss. The dental management is similar to that of children who have leukaemia (see Chapter 50).

Box 49.1 Commonest congenital heart defects in children

Acyanotic
- Ventriculoseptal defect (VSD)
- Atrioseptal defect (ASD)
- Patent ductus arteriosus (PDA)
- Pulmonary stenosis
- Aortic stenosis
- Coarctation of aorta

Cyanotic
- Tetralogy of Fallot (TOF)
- Transposition of great vessels

Box 49.2 Cardiac conditions associated with the highest risk of adverse outcomes from endocarditis

In some countries antibiotic prophylaxis is recommended in patients with the following cardiac conditions if undergoing a specified dental procedure:
- prosthetic cardiac valve or prosthetic material used for cardiac valve repair
- previous infective endocarditis
- congenital heart disease *but* only if it involves:
  - unrepaired cyanotic defects, including palliative shunts and conduits
  - completely repaired defects with prosthetic material or devices, whether placed by surgery or catheter intervention, during the first 6 months after the procedure (after which the prosthetic material is likely to have been endothelialised)
  - repaired defects with residual defects at or adjacent to the site of a prosthetic patch or device (which inhibit endothelialisation)
- cardiac transplantation with the subsequent development of cardiac valvulopathy
- rheumatic heart disease in Indigenous Australians only

Adapted from the Australian guidelines, 2008.

Box 49.3 Recommended antibiotic prophylaxis based on the American and Australian guidelines only for patients at high risk of adverse outcomes from endocarditis

For standard prophylaxis, use:
amoxicillin 2 g (child: 50 mg/kg up to 2 g) orally, 1 hour before the procedure,
or amoxi/ampicillin 2 g (child: 50 mg/kg up to 2 g) IV, just before the procedure,
or amoxi/ampicillin 2 g (child: 50 mg/kg up to 2 g) IM, 30 minutes before the procedure

Patients hypersensitive to penicillin, and those on long-term penicillin therapy or who have taken penicillin or a related beta-lactam antibiotic more than once in the previous month, can use:
clindamycin 600 mg (child: 15 mg/kg up to 600 mg) orally, 1 hour before the procedure or clindamycin 600 mg (child: 15 mg/kg up to 600 mg) IV over at least 20 minutes, just before the procedure
OR
lincomycin 600 mg (child: 15 mg/kg up to 600 mg) IV over at least 1 hour, just before the procedure
OR
vancomycin 25 mg/kg up to 1.5 g (child less than 12 years: 30 mg/kg up to 1.5 g) IV by slow infusion (over at least 60 minutes; rate not exceeding 10 mg/min), ending the infusion just before the procedure
OR
teicoplanin 400 mg (child: 10 mg/kg up to 400 mg) IV, just before the procedure or teicoplanin 400 mg (child: 10 mg/kg up to 400 mg) IM, 30 minutes before the procedure
In case no liquid form of clindamycin is available an alternative for patients who are hypersensitive to penicillin (excluding immediate hypersensitivity), is:
cephalexin 2 g (child: 50 mg/kg up to 2 g) orally, 1 hour before the procedure
Cephalexin is not suitable for those who have been on long-term penicillin or have taken a related beta-lactam antibiotic more than once in the previous month

Paediatric Dentistry at a Glance, First Edition. Monty Duggal, Angus Cameron and Jack Toumba. © 2013 John Wiley & Sons Ltd. Published 2013 by Blackwell Publishing Ltd.

Introduction

Paediatric dentists are required to treat children with heart disease more than any other medically compromised group. Unlike adults most children with heart disease have congenital heart problems. Congenital heart disease (CHD) is seen in 6–8 per 1000 live births with male to female ratio of 1:1. Conditions can be subdivided into cyanotic or acyanotic (Box 49.1). The dental management of this group requires:
- a working knowledge of the various defects and their implications of general health;
- a deep understanding of the impact these have on provision of dental care;
- effective communication with the paediatric cardiology team and paediatric anaesthetist if GA is required;
- a multidisciplinary effort for provision of care.

Dental management

The dental issues that clinicians should consider centre around the safe provision of dental care. Most important are:
- risk of infective endocarditis;
- increased risk of bleeding;
- management under general anaesthesia if required;
- children who require cardiac surgery.

Infective endocarditis (IE)

IE is an infection of the lining of the heart chambers and heart valves caused by bacteria, viruses, fungi or other infectious agents. This can cause growths on the heart valves, the lining of the heart or the lining of blood vessels that may form clots that break off and travel to the brain, lungs, kidneys or spleen.

Dental treatment and IE

Dental treatment is often implicated in the causation of IE. The reason is that although many bacteria can cause IE, *Streptococcus viridans*, which is commonly found in the mouth, is responsible for approximately half of all cases of bacterial endocarditis. Other common organisms include *Staphylococcus* and *Enterococcus*.

Prevention of IE

Opinions have changed recently on the mandatory use of antibiotic (AB) prophylaxis for dental treatment in children with CHD. In the UK for example, the National Institute for Health and Clinical Excellence concluded that there was no evidence of their efficacy; in some countries, including the UK, AB prophylaxis is not used any more for any child with CHD, however "at risk" of endocarditis they might be. In certain countries such as the USA and Australia, there is a move to reconsider the indications and it is used for fewer patients but is still used in children who are believed to be at a greater risk (Box 49.2). The AB prophylaxis protocols that are widely accepted are shown in Box 49.3.

Other measures for prevention of IE

Untreated dental disease in medically compromised children can significantly affect their general health and quality of life. All caries should be treated effectively.
- Pulpally involved teeth should be extracted. Pulp therapy for primary teeth should not be carried out in children with CHD.
- Investigate and treat promptly any dental infections with an antibiotic that covers the organisms that cause IE.
- Endodontic treatment of permanent teeth can and should be carried out. An early establishment of working length and then care to stay within the root canal during preparation should not lead to significant bacteraemia.
- Chlorhexidine mouthwash can be used pre-operatively, although there is no evidence of its efficacy.
- Rigorous prevention and follow-up are required.

Choice of analgesia/anaesthesia

- It is often preferable to avoid subjecting a patient with complex or cyanotic CHD to a general anaesthetic.
- The use of sedation may be useful to reduce the patient's stress.
- An aspirating syringe should be used to give a local anaesthetic if an epinephrine-containing local anaesthetic is used, as the epinephrine may theoretically raise the blood pressure or precipitate dysrhythmias.
- Epinephrine-containing LA can be avoided by using e.g. prilocaine with felypressin instead.
- Adequate analgesia must be provided.
- Gingival retraction cords containing epinephrine should be avoided.
- Interligamentary injection produces a high level of bacteraemia.

Often GA is required, especially for children who would require multiple visits, for which careful preparation of the patient through effective communication with the cardiology team and anaesthetist is required.

Increased risk of bleeding in cyanotic CHD

- Coagulation abnormalities may be seen in cyanotic CHD with secondary polycythaemia, mainly due to chronic hypoxia.
- The patient may be also on anticoagulants such as aspirin or warfarin.
- A full blood count, platelet count, prothrombin time and activated partial thromboplastin time should be performed in cyanotic CHD.
- It is important to avoid dehydrating a cyanotic patient who has secondary polycythaemia.
- Some cardiologists request that a pulse oximeter be used to monitor the cyanotic patient during dental treatment under local anaesthesia as stress and anxiety may lead to rapid desaturation. Emergency equipment must be available at all times.
- The international normalised ratio (INR) is used to monitor the therapeutic effect of an anticoagulant. Where a patient is anticoagulated, the INR should be checked on the day of the procedure to ensure it is at an acceptable level to proceed with treatment.
- Where there are significant abnormalities in screening tests or if a major surgery is planned, treatment may be best carried out in a hospital in consultation with the patient's specialist.

Children requiring cardiac surgery

- Patients who are to undergo cardiac surgery must first have a careful dental evaluation so that any needed dental treatment can be completed beforehand.
- A rigorous preventive programme should be implemented pre- and post-operatively.
- Many cardiologists recommend that dental treatment be avoided in the first 6 months post-operatively where possible as the patient remains at risk of IE for a significant length of time following surgery. Where treatment is unavoidable, the cardiologist should be consulted.

Table 50.1 *Oral effects of cancer treatments.*

Chemotherapy	Radiotherapy

Infections: fungal, viral, *Toxoplasma*, or bacterial
Acute dental infections
Chronic periapical infections can become acute
Ulcers and mucositis
Bleeding and marginal gingivitis, petechiae, ecchymoses, bulla formation
Xerostomia can lead to caries and oral infections
Trismus
Pain in the jaw
Delayed and abnormal development
Septicaemia can be spread from oral infection
	All effects of chemotherapy can also occur with radiotherapy. Specific issues with radiotherapy are:
	   infections
	   radiation caries
	   pulp pain and necrosis
	   tooth hypersensitivity
	   trismus
	   risk of osteoradionecrosis
	   osteomyelitis if bone is affected
	   sialadenitis

Long-term oral effects
Dental abnormalities such as:
   hypoplasia, microdontia
   taurodontism
   failure of teeth to develop
   root constrictions
	Long-term oral effects
	Delayed dental development
	V-shaped roots
	Altered root morphology
	Small crown, incomplete calcification

Box 50.1 Blood indices of which dentists should be aware

Absolute neutrophil count (ANC):
- If $>1 \times 10^{12}$/l – no need for AB prophylaxis; discuss with oncologist
- If $<1 \times 10^{12}$/l – defer elective dental treatment. May need AB prophylaxis and hospitalisation for dental management (AAPD, 2008)

Platelet counts:
- $>50 \times 10^{9}$/l – no additional support needed but may have prolonged bleeding. Local measures or manage with desmopressin (DDAVP) or platelets
- $<50 \times 10^{9}$/l – defer dental treatment. In dental emergency, contact oncologist. Platelets required for any surgery procedure (Scully and Cawson, 2005)

Box 50.2 Suggested methods for improving oral comfort during cancer therapy

Mucositis: palliative treatment of symptoms. Use of topical LA
Oral mucosal infections: check and treat for fungal, viral and bacterial infections
Fungal infections: topical nystatin not used. Systemic antifungals if positive culture
Oral culture/biopsies of all suspicious lesions
Oral bleeding: occurs due to thrombocytopenia, disturbance in clotting factors and damaged vascular integrity. May need antifibrinolytic rinses, or systemic measures (platelet transfusion, aminocaproic acid)
Dental sensitivity/pain: related to decreased secretion of saliva and lowered salivary pH. Patients who are using vincristine may present with pain, mostly in the mandible, in the absence of any obvious pathology, which resolves with discontinuation of the drug
Xerostomia: sugar-free chewing gum, special dentifrices for oral dryness, saliva substitutes, frequent sipping of water, and alcohol-free oral rinses
Fluoride rinses and varnishes are strongly recommended for caries prevention
Trismus: particularly radiotherapy involving jaws. Seek help from maxillofacial colleagues

Paediatric Dentistry at a Glance, First Edition. Monty Duggal, Angus Cameron and Jack Toumba. © 2013 John Wiley & Sons Ltd. Published 2013 by Blackwell Publishing Ltd.

Introduction

The paediatric dentist plays an important role in diagnosis, prevention, stabilisation and treatment of the oral and dental problems that can compromise the child's quality of life before, during and after cancer treatment. It is essential to have an understanding of the impact of the condition and its treatment on the child's general heath, and the implications of oral health and comfort, and provision of dental treatment.

Treatment of childhood cancers

A combination of the following treatments is used: chemotherapy, radiotherapy, surgery and bone marrow/stem cell transplantation with or without total body irradiation. Chemotherapy and radiotherapy can have profound impact on oral tissues (Table 50.1) and also on provision of dental care.

Issues that need to be considered by dentists

• The child has been diagnosed with a life-threatening condition. An empathetic approach is required.

• Some forms of cancer may, and frequently do, have oral manifestations.

• The cancer, in particular those involving the haemopoietic tissues, may lead to the child's immune system being compromised (direct immune suppression).

• Most treatment protocols causes indirect immune suppression which can be severe and will have implications for dental treatment (Table 50.1).

• Many treatment protocols for the cancer cause oral side-effects.

Dental management for children with cancer

1. Before the initiation of cancer therapy: at diagnosis.
2. During immunosuppression periods: during treatment.
3. After the cancer therapy is completed: in remission.

Before initiation of cancer therapy

This should involve three steps:

1. Initial oral assessment including radiographs if possible. Diagnosis and treatment protocol are noted.

2. Preventive advice within the context of the patient's and family's stressful situation is provided with sensitivity and empathy.

3. Essential dental treatment that must be completed before cancer therapy is planned. This includes:

  • removal of teeth likely to be a source of infection when child is immune suppressed: extractions should be completed at least 7 days before start of chemotherapy in order to allow healing;

  • dressing and stabilising teeth that can be restored once remission is achieved.

During acute phase of treatment and immune suppression

Five to 7 days after the beginning of each cycle of chemotherapy the blood count starts falling, staying low for 14–21 days, before rising again to normal levels for a few days until the next cycle begins. Only emergency dental treatment should be provided in this stage. Emphasis is on improving oral comfort from oral side-effects due to direct stomatoxicity of the drug or indirect effects through immune suppression (Table 50.1). It is important for dentists to understand what the threshold of the blood indices are for safe delivery of dental treatment (Box 50.1). All efforts should be made to provide supportive oral care for the child to improve oral comfort during cancer treatment (Box 50.2).

During remission and discharge

• Active monitoring and rigorous prevention are required.

• Radiotherapy to oral tissues will lead to xerostomia requiring intensive prevention. Toothpastes containing high concentrations of fluoride (2800/5000 ppm) are useful as is Tooth Mousse (GC).

• Restorative care and extractions can be safely provided but check blood indices first. For those who had radiotherapy involving the jaws, liaise with the oncologist to prevent osteoradionecrosis.

• For those who have received high-dose radiation to the jaws, hyperbaric oxygen and high-dose antibiotic prophylaxis may be required prior to extraction surgery involving oral hard tissues.

Dental management specific to bone marrow transplantation

General principles are the same as described above. Pre-transplant conditioning and the post-transplant therapies cause prolonged immunosuppression following the transplant. Elective dentistry needs to be postponed until immunological recovery, to at least 9–12 months after stem cell transplantation, and longer if the patient has chronic graft-versus-host disease (GVHD) or other complications. It is important to screen patients and complete all essential dental treatment before transplantation is carried out. A good relationship with the transplant team is required. Most transplant recipients will be on long-term immune suppressive therapies which has implications for dental treatment.

Long-term dental impact on survivors of childhood cancer

Cancer treatment targets rapidly dividing cancer cells but damage to other cells that might be dividing rapidly at the time is inevitable. Tooth germ is no exception and many long-term survivors have defects affecting the permanent teeth. The most severe defects are reported for children who have had radiotherapy involving the jaws, In these cases the long-term defects reported are: hypoplastic teeth; arrested root development or complete or partial root aplasia; long-lasting xerostomia, predisposing to development of severe form of rampant caries, also known as radiation caries; long-term risk of developing osteoradionecrosis.

Table 51.1 Diabetic emergencies. Data from Scully and Cawson, 2005 and McKenna, 2006.

	Hypoglycaemia	Hyperglycaemia
Cause	Excess insulin Missed meals Overexertion/exercise Anxiety	Relative or absolute deficiency of insulin
Symptoms and presentation	Rapid onset Irritability Disorientation Blurred vision Slurred speech Hypothermia Tachycardia Warm sweaty skin Dilated pupils Anxiety Loss of consciousness	Slow onset Dry skin and mouth Weak pulse Hypotension Hyperventilation Acetone smell on breath Vomiting Loss of consciousness
Management	Measure blood glucose levels Give 15 g of glucose drink, tablets or gel If unconscious or uncooperative, give 1 mg glucagon IM (for children <5 years, give 0.5 mg). Another alternative is 50 ml of 50% dextrose IV If recovery is delayed, the emergency services should be called	Measure blood glucose levels Establish IV infusion of 80% bicarbonate Obtain medical opinion If there is any doubt about the diagnosis, glucose should be administered as a diagnostic test. This will cause no harm in the hyperglycaemic individual

Table 51.2 Effect of oral disease on health of diabetic children.

Oral disease	Effect on general health
Periodontal disease	Chronic periodontal infection may contribute to hyperglycaemia and treatment of infection reduces the percentage of glycosylated haemoglobin
Acute dental oral infections	Acute infection induces metabolic changes particularly in carbohydrate metabolism and affects diabetic control • Liaise with paediatricians for glucose control • Identify source of infection and treat aggressively

Paediatric Dentistry at a Glance, First Edition. Monty Duggal, Angus Cameron and Jack Toumba. © 2013 John Wiley & Sons Ltd. Published 2013 by Blackwell Publishing Ltd.

Diabetes mellitus

This is a common condition affecting at least 2% of the British population and up to 6% of the population of the USA. It encompasses a group of metabolic disorders characterised by chronic hyperglycaemia resulting from defects in insulin secretion, insulin action or both.

Types affecting children

• **Type 1 diabetes mellitus** (insulin-dependent diabetes mellitus, IDDM); also known as juvenile-onset diabetes, accounting for 5% of all cases.
• **Type 2 diabetes mellitus** (non-insulin-dependent diabetes mellitus, NIDDM); also known as maturity-onset diabetes, type 2 accounts for 95% of all cases of diabetes mellitus. Onset is usually in mid or later life, although it can occur earlier. It develops mainly through a combination of insulin resistance and defective B-cell function. It may remain asymptomatic until diagnosed by a routine blood or urine test.
• **Maturity-onset diabetes of youth** (MODY), a rare, inherited form of type 2 diabetes that usually affects teenagers.

Blood glucose range

The normal blood glucose level is 3.9–6.1 mmol/l.

WHO range of blood glucose indicative of diabetes mellitus is as follows:
• fasting plasma glucose (FPG) ≥7.0 mmol/l;
• plasma glucose ≥11.1 mmol/l at 2 hours after a 75 g oral glucose load (oral glucose tolerance test, OGTT).

Dental management

The following advice mainly applies to IDDM. The main concern about treating people with diabetes is their potential for collapse due to hypoglycaemia and, less commonly, hyperglycaemia. Diabetic emergencies are summarised in Table 51.1. The effect of untreated oral disease on diabetes is shown in Table 51.2.

Routine dental treatment

• Dental appointments should be short and as stress, pain and trauma free as possible as anxiety can increase blood glucose levels.
• Early morning appointments are least likely to interfere with the diabetes control regime. They have also been advocated because endogenous corticosteroids levels tend to be higher, allowing better tolerance of stressful procedures.
• People with well controlled diabetes (who are otherwise fit) can have general dental treatment and minor oral surgery carried out under local anaesthesia, inhalation sedation or IV sedation in general dental practice, provided that their normal regime of food, drugs or insulin is not disturbed.
• Appointments should be timed so that they do not interfere with the drug and diet regime.

• Patients should be advised to adhere to their normal patterns of medication and diet control to minimise the risk of hypoglycaemia.
• A good medical history including the diabetes treatment regime and stability of control is important. Patients should be asked about any previous episodes of hyper- or hypoglycaemic attacks.
• Patient should be asked to tell the treating dentist if they feel unwell or if they can feel a hypoglycaemic attack starting.
• Drugs such as aspirin, steroids and levofloxacin should be avoided. Levofloxacin can cause hypoglycaemia and enhance the effect of oral hypoglycaemic agents.
• Local anaesthesia can usually be used safely and most anaesthetic drugs are safe for use in these patients.

For surgical procedures

Avoid hypoglycaemia but keep hyperglycaemia below levels that may be harmful because of delayed wound healing or phagocyte dysfunction. The desired whole blood glucose levels are 3–5 mmol/l (120–180 mg/dl).

In a well controlled diabetic, providing that normal diet can be taken and normal antidiabetic drugs are not interrupted, minor surgical procedures such as single tooth extraction can be safely carried out.

Dental management under GA

This may be complicated by hypoglycaemia or associated complications such as chronic renal failure, ischaemic heart disease or neuropathy, which carries a risk of cardiorespiratory arrest under general anaesthesia. Stress and trauma raise insulin requirements and precipitate ketoacidosis. Close liaison with the paediatrician is required.
• Pre-operative assessment: the patient should be put on soluble insulin and stabilised. Control should be confirmed by estimation of blood sugar (fasting, midday and before the evening meal).
• The procedure should be carried out early in the morning and booked first in the list, so that any delays in the operation schedule will not impair diabetic control.
• First thing in the morning, blood should be taken for glucose estimation and intravenous infusion set up giving glucose 10 g, soluble insulin 2 units and potassium 2 mmol/h, until normal oral feeding is resumed, at which time the patient can be returned to the pre-operative insulin regimen.
• Blood glucose should be monitored at 2–4-hourly intervals until the patient is feeding normally.
• The endocrinologist or physician should be consulted for uncontrolled diabetics or those requiring a long operation under GA.

Antibiotic cover

Routine administration of prophylactic antibiotic to prevent post-operative infection should be considered only in situations where they would be used for non-diabetic patients. Some advocate the use of antibiotics in poorly controlled diabetics who need emergency invasive treatment, such as extractions.

Kidney and liver disease and organ transplantation

Box 52.1 Possible oral effects of kidney disease

Enamel hypoplasia

Predentine changes – thickened predentine layer

Decreased levels of dental caries:
- Increased salivary pH due to urea/ammonia
- Reduced *Streptococcus mutans* levels

Salivary pH and buffering capacity:
- Increased pH
- Increased buffering capacity

Gingival health:
- Gingival overgrowth
- Uraemic stomatitis
- Petechiae
- Ecchymoses

Changes in oral microflora

Bone metabolism:
- Demineralisation of the jaw bones, "ground glass" appearance
- Loss of lamina dura
- Localised radiolucent jaw lesions
- Loss of trabeculation
- Giant cell lesions
- Delayed eruption
- Pulp calcifications
- Bony fractures and bone tumours secondary to hyperparathyroidism may occur

Oral malodour/bad taste

Box 52.2 Possible oral effects of liver disease

Haemorrhage:
- Petechiae
- Haematoma
- Jaundiced mucosal tissues
- Gingival bleeding
- Reduced healing after surgery

Bilirubin pigmentation of teeth: green discolouration

Increased risk of dental caries

Gingival hypertrophy

Delayed eruption

Enamel hypoplasia

Box 52.3 Possible oral manifestations of GVHD

Sicca syndrome

Depapillation of the tongue with variegations

Scalloping of lateral margins

Lichen planus

Oral ulcers

Angular tightness

Paediatric Dentistry at a Glance, First Edition. Monty Duggal, Angus Cameron and Jack Toumba. © 2013 John Wiley & Sons Ltd. Published 2013 by Blackwell Publishing Ltd.

Kidney disease

The incidence of end-stage renal failure (ESRF) in childhood, either due to a congenital or acquired condition is roughly 10–12 per 1 million children. As for many other chronic childhood illnesses, significant improvements in dialysis and organ transplantation have meant that many children are long-term survivors and, consequently, dentists will be required to provide dental treatment for such children who have either chronic renal failure (CRF), ESRF, or are recipients of renal transplant. Dentists should be aware of two issues:

• oral and dental implications as these conditions have a multi-organ implication (Box 52.1);
• implications of the disease and its treatment for provision of dental care.

Dental management

• Liaise with the child's named paediatrician.
• Check blood indices, in particular the coagulation parameters before invasive dental treatment.
• Adjustment of the dose of several drugs is required due to the kidneys' reduced ability for metabolism and secretion. For example, the dose of midazolam must be reduced by 50% in patients with a glomerular filtration rate (GFR) <10 ml/min/1.73 m², check with the paediatrician before making any adjustments.
• Prescription of systemic fluorides is avoided because of the decreased renal clearance of fluoride, and these patients' low susceptibility to dental caries.
• Any dental infection should be treated aggressively, keeping in mind the required antibiotic dosage.
• For patients undergoing haemodialysis, procedures involving bleeding or requiring antibiotic prophylaxis should not be carried out on the day of dialysis. If the patient has an arteriovenous fistula or central line, they may require antibiotic prophylaxis, please use national guidelines as these may vary from country to country. Blood pressure cuff or IV medications should not be administered into the shunt arm. Heparinisation may put these patients at risk of prolonged bleeding.
• All potential or present foci of infection should be removed as a part of the essential pre-transplant preparation of the patient.
• Post-transplantation, always consult the paediatric nephrologist about the transplant function and the degree of immunosuppression. Steroid and/or antibiotic cover will be required in many cases. Regular review is required. Gingival hyperplasia may occur in patients taking cyclosporin. Inform the nephrologist who could substitute this with tacrolimus which does not have this side-effect.

Liver disease

The following are the most commonly occurring diseases affecting the liver in children:

• hepatitis A, B, C, D or E;
• autoimmune hepatitis;
• haemochromatosis;
• Wilson's disease.

Dental management

Disorders of the liver have many implications for a patient receiving dental treatment (Box 52.2). Dentists should be aware of the potential for increased bleeding as well as drug toxicity. Prior to liver transplantation, treat potential sources of infection aggressively. Preventive care is important before and after transplantation. High-speed suction has been advocated during dental procedures to prevent ingestion of blood, as it is metabolised by the liver. Antibiotic prophylaxis and/or steroid cover may be required for certain procedures.

Bleeding tendency

Liver disease may result in depressed plasma levels of coagulation factors. Check blood indices including a full blood count, prothrombin time, activated partial thromboplastin time, INR, bleeding time, and liver function tests. If any abnormal levels are discovered, consultation with the hepatologist is important before beginning dental treatment. If oral surgical procedures are required, minimise trauma to the patient. If there is a significant risk of bleeding an infusion of fresh frozen plasma may be indicated. Advanced oral surgical procedures or any dental procedures in a patient with a coagulopathy may need to be carried out in a hospital setting.

Reduction of drug dosage

Certain sedatives (diazepam, barbiturates) and general anaesthetics (halothane) can impair detoxification in hepatic disease and should be used cautiously. Brain metabolism may be altered, and sensitivity to medications may increase. Caution should be used in prescribing medications metabolised in the liver, such as isoniazid, non-steroidal anti-inflammatory agents, phenytoin, phenobarbital, valproic acid and some sulfonamides.

Local anaesthetics should be administered cautiously to patients with hepatic impairment. Most amides are primarily metabolised in the liver and therefore may reach toxic levels with lower doses of anaesthetic. Articaine (plasma) and prilocaine (partly in lungs), however, have other sites of metabolism. Drug dosages and possible interactions should be discussed with a treating physician. In some cases, lower drug dosages are required, while some drugs (erythromycin, metronidazole, tetracyclines) should be avoided completely. Non-steroidal anti-inflammatory agents should be used cautiously or avoided due to an increased risk of gastrointestinal bleeding and interference with fluid balance.

Organ transplantation

Although **syngeneic** transplantation does not usually pose a significant immunological risk, **allogenic** transplantation presents two key problems:

• genetic variation between donor and recipient;
• immunological recognition of the variation.

This leads to acute and chronic graft versus host disease (GVHD). See Box 52.3.

Consult responsible physician. Consider bleeding tendency, risk of infection and impaired drug metabolism. The patient may need steroid supplementation and cover for up to 2 years post transplant. It is best to defer elective dental treatment until at least 3 months after transplant. Certain drugs, as above, should be used with caution.

53 Prescribing drugs for children

Table 53.1 a–f Doses of some most commonly used drugs used by dental professionals for children. Data from British National Formulary for Children 2011–2012.

(a)

Drug	1m–1 year	1–6 years	6–12 years	12–18 years
Penicillin V	62.5 mg 4 times/day Increased up to 12.5 mg/kg 4 times/day in severe infections	125 mg 4 times/day Increased up to 12.5 mg/kg 4 times/day in severe infections	250 mg 4 times/day Increased up to 12.5 mg/kg 4 times/day in severe infections	500 mg 4 times/day Increased up to 1g 4 times/day in severe infections

(b)

Drug	1m–1 year	1–5 years	5–18 years
Amoxicillin	62.5 mg 3 times/day Dose doubled in severe infections	125 mg 3 times/day Dose doubled in severe infections	250 mg 3 times/day Dose doubled in severe infections

(c)

Drug	1m–2 years	2–8 years	8–18 years
Erythromycin	125 mg 4 times/day, doubled in severe infections	250 mg 4 times/day, doubled in severe infections	250–500 mg 4 times/day, doubled in severe infections

(d)

Drug	1–3 years	3–7 years	7–10 years	10–18 years
Metronidazole	50 mg every 8 hours	100 mg every 12 hours	100 mg every 8 hours	200–250 mg every 8 hours

(e)

Drug	1–6 years	6–12 years	12–18 years
Paracetamol			
For pain with or without pyrexia	120–250 mg every 4–6 hours Max 4 doses in 24 hours	250–500 mg every 4–6 hours Max 4 doses in 24 hours	500 mg every 4–6 hours
For post-operative pain	20–30 mg/kg followed by 15–20 mg/kg every 4–6 hours Max 90 mg/kg in 24 hours in divided doses	20–30 mg/kg (1g max) followed by 15–20 mg/kg every 4–6 hours Max 90 mg/kg in 24 hours in divided doses	1g every 4–6 hours Max 4 doses in 24 hours

(f)

Drug	6m–1 year	1–4 years	4–7 years	7–10 years	10–12 years	12–18 years
Ibuprofen	50 mg 3–4 times/day Max 30 mg/kg in 3–4 divided doses daily	100 mg 3 times/day Max 30 mg/kg in 3–4 divided doses daily	150 mg 3 times/day Max 30 mg/kg in 3–4 divided doses daily	200 mg 3 times/day Max 30 mg/kg (max 2.4 g) in 3–4 divided doses daily	300 mg 3 times/day Max 30 mg/kg (max 2.4 g) in 3–4 divided doses daily	300–400 mg 3–4 times/day increased to max 600 mg 4 times/day if necessary

Paediatric Dentistry at a Glance, First Edition. Monty Duggal, Angus Cameron and Jack Toumba. © 2013 John Wiley & Sons Ltd. Published 2013 by Blackwell Publishing Ltd.

Introduction

Medicines should only be given to children when they are absolutely necessary and after a careful evaluation of the risk–benefit. Most children who attend a dental practice with toothache do not require antibiotics, as in most situations pain can be managed with local measures. Antibiotics should not be prescribed unless there is a good indication that the patient has infection with systemic effects as opposed to pain from pulpitis. Children differ from adults in their response to drugs and doses should always be calculated carefully. Children who are on long-term medication for medical conditions should be given oral health advice, especially those where the medicines contain cariogenic sugars. Wherever possible, medical personnel should be encouraged to use sugar-free options.

Prescription writing

Local guidelines should be followed but some important principles of prescription writing are:
- legible writing with indelible ink;
- patient's age, date of birth and address should be included;
- name of drug clearly written and not abbreviated;
- form, e.g. tablets, suspension etc., should be specified;
- dose, dose frequency and interval should be clearly stated; consider including the dose/kg body weight for pharmacist to double check;
- quantity to be supplied to the patient;
- name and signature of the prescriber.

Calculating dose for children

In most authoritative texts on the subject such as the British National Formulary (BNF), doses are standardised according to the body weight. The weight standardised dose is multiplied by the child's weight. However the dose calculated in this way should not normally exceed the maximum recommended for an adult, so for children who are very overweight, ideal weight and height should be used.

Drug preparation

The ability of the child to swallow tablets or capsules should be assessed as should the child's preference. Poor compliance can result from giving the child the wrong preparation. Clear instructions on the amount, and frequency of dosage should be given to the carers of very young children. Sometimes if the dosing is not in simple multiples of 5 ml, an oral syringe for accurate measurement of the amount is given to the parent.

Prescribing in children with co-morbidities

Children with liver disease

Modification of the choice and dose of the drugs is required occasionally especially in the following situations:
- liver failure, special precautions with certain drugs such as sedatives;
- impaired coagulation, might alter effects of anticoagulants;
- drugs with known hepatotoxicity. If hepatic impairment is suspected or known consult the physician. Some drugs used in dental practice, such as flucloxacillin, will need careful consideration for use in hepatic impairment.

Children with renal impairment

Drug prescribing should be avoided in children with renal disease. If renal impairment is suspected consult the physician, as renal function might need to be checked before any dose modification. Some drugs used in dental practice, such as penicillin G and amoxicillin, will need to be avoided or their doses modified in children with renal impairment. Drugs with known nephrotoxicity are avoided in these children as the nephrotoxicity will be enhanced in children with renal impairment.

Adverse reaction to drugs

In children never use any drug unless there is a clear indication for so doing. As few drugs are prescribed as possible and it is best practice to use drugs that are familiar. Careful history should be taken to ensure that the child has no known allergies to the drugs being prescribed. Carers should be clearly instructed to report any effects immediately to the prescriber and discontinue the drug if they suspect any adverse reaction to it.

If any side-effects are reported the drug is discontinued immediately and this is clearly recorded in the patient's records. It is also the duty of all health professionals to report any side effects of drugs to whichever national body in their country keeps such records.

Commonly used antibiotics and analgesics in dental practice

The doses of the drugs mentioned below are given in Table 53.1.

Antibiotics

- **Phenoxymethyl penicillin (Pen V), amoxicillin.** These are usually the first-choice antibiotics for dental infections. Amoxicillin has an advantage as it is taken 3 times/day which is easier to manage for children.

For those who are allergic to penicillin:
- **Erythromycin.** This has a similar antibacterial spectrum to penicillin.
- **Metronidazole.** This is used for anaerobic infections and also in combination with amoxicillin in severe orofacial infections with systemic symptoms.

Analgesics

- **Paracetamol.** This is the first choice but has no anti-inflammatory effects. It causes hepatotoxicity in high doses.
- **Ibuprofen.** This is used for moderate pain and inflammation. It must not be used in children with gastrointestinal ulceration.

References

American Academy of Pediatric Dentistry (2008) Guideline on Dental Management of Paediatric Patients Receiving Chemotherapy, Hematopoietic Cell Transplantation, and/or Radiation. Available on the World Wide Web <http://www.aapd.org/media/Policies_Guidelines/G_Chemo.pdf> Pp. 219–225. (Accessed on 5 June 2009).

American Academy of Pediatric Dentistry Clinical Affairs Committee – Behavior Management Subcommittee (2008) Guideline on behavior guidance for the pediatric dental patient. Pediatric Dentistry 2008:30 (7 Suppl): 125–133.

Bowlby, J. (1969) *Attachment and Loss, Vol. 1: Attachment*. New York: Basic Books.

British National Formulary for Children (2011–2012) London: Pharmaceutical Press. www.bnfc.org

Duggal, M.S., Curzon, M.E.J., Fayle, S.A., Toumba, K.J. and Robertson, A.J. (2002) *Restorative Techniques in Pediatric Dentistry. An Illustrated Guide to the Restoration of Carious Primary Teeth*, 2nd edn. London: Martin Dunitz Publishers.

Duggal M.S., Nooh A, High, AS (2002). Response of the primary pulp to inflammation: a review of the Leeds studies and challenges for the future. Eur J Paediatr Dent 3: 111–114.

Feigal, R.J. (2001) Guiding and managing the child dental patient: a fresh look at old pedagogy. J Dent Educ 65(12): 1369–1377.

Freeman, R. (1999) The case for mother in the surgery. Brit Dent J 186: 610–613.

Guidelines on the use of Dental Radiographs. www.eapd.eu

Kassa D, Day P, High A, Duggal MS (2008). Histological comparison of pulpal inflammation in primary teeth with occlusal or proximal caries. Int J Paed Dent 19: 23–26.

Lowrey, G.H. (1973) *Growth and Development of Children*. Chicago: Year Book Medical Publishers, Inc.

McDonagh, M.S., Whiting, P.F., Wilson, P.M., Sutton, A.J., Chestnutt, I., Cooper, J., Misso, K., Bradley, M., Treasure, E. and Kleijnen, J. (2000) Systematic review of water fluoridation. BMJ 321: 855–859.

McKenna, S.J. (2006) Dental management of patients with diabetes. Dent Clin North Am 50: 591–606.

Ravn, J.J. (1981) Follow-up study of permanent incisors with enamel cracks as result of an acute trauma. Scand J Dent Res 89: 117–123.

Research, Science and Therapy Committee, American Academy of Periodontology (2003) Periodontal diseases of children and adolescents. J Periodontol 74: 1696–1704.

Scully, C. and Cawson, R.A. (2005) *Medical Problems in Dentistry*, 5th edn. Edinburgh: Elsevier Churchill Livingstone.

Teasdale, G. and Jennett, B. (1974) Assessment of coma and impaired consciousness: a practical scale. Lancet 304: 81–84.

Toumba, K.J. and Lygidakis, N.A. (2009) Guidelines on the use of fluoride in children: an EAPD policy document. Eur Arch Paediatr Dent 10: 129–135. www.eapd.eu

Wolpe, J. (1969) *The Practice of Behavior Therapy*. New York: Pergamon Press.

Wright, G.Z. and Alpern, G.D. (1971) Variables influencing children's co-operative behavior at first dental visit. J Dent Child 23: 124–128.

Index

Note: page numbers in *italics* refer to figures, and those in **bold** refer to tables or boxed material.

Paediatric Dentistry at a Glance, First Edition. Monty Duggal, Angus Cameron and Jack Toumba. © 2013 John Wiley & Sons Ltd. Published 2013 by Blackwell Publishing Ltd.

tuberous sclerosis   81
tumours, jaw and soft tissues   75, 85

ulceration, oral   78–9
uncomplicated fractures
   permanent teeth   *62,* 63, 69
   primary teeth   61

vancomycin   **102**
vesiculobullous lesions   78–9
viral infections   79, 81

visual inspection, caries   36–7
vitamin D-resistant rickets   93
Vitapex   47
voice modulation   12
vomiting   39
von Willebrand's disease   99
Vygotsky's sociocultural theory   11

Wand   15, *16,* 17
ward staff, communication with   21
warfarin   99

warts, viral   81
water fluoridation   33
white spot lesions   *34,* 35, 41

xerostomia *see* dry mouth

zinc oxide eugenol   47